I0417964

# DREAMS OF SANITY

A Journey of Depression and Beyond

ANITA PLACIDO

Copyright © 2025 Anita Placido

ISBN: 979-8-218-67617-9

All rights reserved. No part of this book may be used or reproduced by any means, graphic, electronic, or mechanical, including photocopying, recording, taping or by any information storage retrieval system without the written permission of the author except in the case of brief quotations embodied in critical articles and reviews.

Scriptures taken from the Holy Bible, New International Version®, NIV®. Copyright © 1973, 1978, 1984, 2011 by Biblica, Inc.™ Used by permission of Zondervan. All rights reserved worldwide. www.zondervan.com The "NIV" and "New International Version" are trademarks registered in the United States Patent and Trademark Office by Biblica, Inc.™

You Are A Child Of Mine Words and Music by Christopher Eaton and Mark Schultz Copyright © 2003 Here's To Jo Music, West Lodge Music and Crazy Romaine Music All Rights for Here's To Jo Music and West Lodge Music Administered by BMG Rights Management (US) LLC All Rights for Crazy Romaine Music Administered by Music Services All Rights Reserved Used by Permission Reprinted by Permission of Hal Leonard LLC

This book is dedicated to my wonderful family, Nick, Sarah, Jack, Miriam, and José, who have loved me, cared for me, stood by me, and supported me on this long, difficult journey;

and to Mark, who allowed himself to be a vessel used by God to bring healing. I am so grateful for his help and guidance to find my "new normal."

May God richly bless you!

# Contents

# Acknowledgements

The author wishes to thank the following people for their assistance, insight, direction, and encouragement in the writing of this book: Mark, my therapist, who started the whole process of my healing; my initial concept readers, Abby, Bonnie, Diana, and Linda; my proofreaders, Linda and Kelly; and Judy, who helped put it into the right format and did a super job editing; and most of all my loving husband, Nick, for his support and encouragement, and my children, Sarah, Jack, Miriam, and José for their help along the journey to a healthy life.

# Preface

This is my story of how God brought me through a dark time of depression in my life and His ever-surprising methods of bringing reconciliation and healing. It is important for me to tell you that I still struggle at times with mild depression due to Seasonal Affective Disorder and a chemical imbalance. Although I have adopted lifestyle changes of consistent sleep patterns, a healthier diet, and exercise, I still take a low dose of medication. There are times when life can be somewhat overwhelming; I do not want you to think I have arrived and am free from depression. It is merely that I have learned and continue to learn how to cope appropriately with the challenges life presents, as you will see later in the book, instead of falling back into the negative patterns that brought me to the point where I could no longer keep up my defenses against the depression. I now know that I must trust God to give me the strength and wisdom to make good choices in my life.

Because my story talks about my experience of sexual abuse at a young age and a difficult living arrangement when I was a little older, some of this book will deal with the issues of sex and intimacy. I do not wish to offend anyone, but this was a major piece of my life that contributed to my depression and it shows how God took even those horrible situations and used them for His glory. God showed me that I had a choice of whether or not I let those memories and events rule my life. It doesn't make them any less real, but now when I think of them I just feel sad that they happened. God has healed the anger and fear that used to control my thoughts and actions.

My desire for this book is that it will be a source of hope and encouragement to those suffering from depression and to those who are suffering from the emotional scars of abuse. I hope it can also be of help to those who have friends or family members dealing with these situations.

I recognize God works differently in the lives of everyone and uses their unique personalities, experiences and circumstances in a way that speaks directly to them to bring His healing. This is my story of the unique ways He worked in my life to bring me back to Himself and free me from things that were hindering my ability to cope with everyday life. I pray that you will seek Him and be open to however He chooses to work in your life.

# 1

# Background with Daddy

In order for the following chapters to make sense, you need to know some of the events in my early life that shaped the unhealthy coping mechanisms that got me through my life for forty-one years. In October 2003, I could no longer keep the buried emotions at bay through my regular methods, and the walls I built up came crashing down.

I am an only child, born to parents who had tried for years to have children. By the time I finally arrived, my father was thirty-nine and my mother was thirty-two years old.

From stories I have heard about my dad's life before I was born, he was a wonderful and smart man. He graduated at the top of his class in business school. Unfortunately, he graduated during the Great Depression and financial jobs were hard to find. He loved to travel and see new things. Before I was born, my parents went on a three-week vacation across South Dakota, Montana, Wyoming, and on to Yellowstone and Yosemite National Parks. They also took an extended vacation around the entire state of Florida, down the east coast, then to the Keys, and up the west coast. He used to tell my mom that if she saw something she wanted to visit, she should say so and they would stop because "he might not be coming back this way again." I believe at some point he was crushed by the circumstances and disappointments of his life and began a downward spiral.

When I was about ten months old, my father left my mom and me and moved out to Arizona. A few months after he left, my mom took me and followed him there. We stayed there a couple of years while he worked for Lockheed. A transfer with Lockheed took us to another state. We had lived there about a year when my dad discovered that my mom was trying to get a job back where we lived when I was born. He told her to go back, but she could not take me with her. He did not really want me there, but that was her punishment for leaving. So she left, and I lived with him for two more years. They never did divorce.

I don't remember very much of those early years. I believe God in His mercy and grace blocked out a lot of my memories from that time. I do know I was sexually molested when I was around four years old. It was not a single incident but rather a recurring situation. I never told anyone because I didn't know that what was happening to me was not normal.

One night I had been with other kids while they were riding their bikes. I didn't have a bike, so one of the girls put me on her handlebars and we rode around the neighborhood. My foot slipped and went into the spokes of the bike. It broke my leg just above the ankle and the fibula bone was sticking out of my leg. I was so afraid to tell my dad what happened that I put my sock and shoe back on and went back to the house. My dad was sitting at the kitchen table. I managed to walk as normally as possible past them and went to my room. I went to bed, but in the middle of the night my leg hurt so bad that I was crying loudly. My dad came in to see what was wrong. When he saw my leg he took me to the hospital. They reset the bone and put my leg in a cast. A month later he put me on a plane to go back to live with my mom.

I know my time living with him was not all good because when I arrived at my mom's at age five, I only weighed twenty-five pounds and I was severely malnourished. When I got off the plane in my cast, my mom cried because I was dirty. I had on a threadbare dress and my hair was a wild mass of tangles matted with mucus.

When I went back to my mom, I never saw or heard from my dad again. He died at age forty-nine of a massive heart attack when I was ten years old.

# 2

# Background with
# Mom and Ben

L et me begin this chapter by saying that my mother was a great mom during most of my time with her from five years old until I went off to college. She was very creative and would help me and my friends make cookies or Christmas cards and ornaments. She was the mom in the neighborhood who always made snacks for my friends, the "Kool-Aid Mom." When I came home from school, she would have a snack and we would talk about my day. She was a professional seamstress and worked out of our house, making most of my clothes until I was in high school. She really did a great job as a mom in most areas. However, in one aspect, her living arrangement and actions had a profound effect on me as I grew up.

When I returned to my mom from living with my dad, there was a man with her when she picked me up at the airport. He was introduced to me as "Ben," although that was not his real name. Mom never explained who he was or why he was there.

As I grew up, I knew that Mom loved me and would take care of me the best she could, but there were times that made me question what would happen to me if she were forced to choose between me and Ben. She had already made that choice once before when she left me to live with my dad.

Mom and I lived in an apartment paid for by Ben, but he did not live there with us. He never stayed overnight. When I was seven years old he bought a house for us out in the suburbs.

After we moved to the suburbs, I used to come to my mom's room in the middle of the night and stand by her bed, just staring at her. She would wake up and ask what was wrong, but I wouldn't answer her. I was sleepwalking. I had been abandoned once by each parent and, subconsciously, I was checking to make sure she was still there. She would tell me everything was okay and to go back to bed.

When I was around eight years old, I woke up and heard noises in the house. I opened my door and heard my mom making sounds like she was being hurt. I called her name and she yelled at me to get back in bed. For several nights I would lie on the floor and listen under my door. I was both curious and terrified. I did not know what was going on (although when I got older I realized they were having sex),

5

and I was afraid she was in danger. What would happen to me if I lost her, too?

After several nights of listening to them, I could not handle the fear any more. I wrote a note and slipped it in my mom's pocket when she wasn't looking. It said, "If you don't stop what you two are doing, I'm going to drink the Drano." Although it sounded like a suicide threat, I am sure I would have never actually carried it out. It was a cry for help to understand what was happening and to be reassured that she was okay. If she had just said that it was the way two people expressed their love to each other and no one was hurt, I would have been fine and dropped it. But that was not her reaction. She found the note and came to me asking what it was about. I told her I was afraid she was being hurt and I was scared of losing her. Her response was, "That is a bunch of foolishness. I don't ever want to hear about this again," and she walked away. That was when I got the message that my feelings were not important and I should not bring them up or talk about them. I retreated even further behind the emotional wall I had built to shield myself during the molestation when I was younger.

One afternoon when I was in junior high, I came home from school and ran in to tell my mom something exciting that happened that day. I burst into her bedroom and found them having sex. They both started screaming at me to get out. I ran outside, not understanding what I had seen. I sat on our back porch until my mom came and told me to come in. Ben had left and nothing was ever said about it. From that day on, though, the front door of our house was locked when I came home from school and I had to sit on the front porch, where the neighbors could see me, and wait until they came and opened the door. When they opened it, it was like nothing out of the ordinary was happening. My mom would ask how my day was at school. I would just go to my room and not answer her. Inside I was angry. They knew what time I got home from school every day. Why couldn't they have sex before I got home? Why was I the one being locked out? But I could never say anything like that out loud to either one of them. I knew to keep my feelings to myself.

When deer season opened, Mom and Ben always went deer hunting for a week. My birthday was always near the opening day of hunting season, so they were never home for my birthday my entire childhood, thus reinforcing the message I perceived from them that I was not of worth or value. I was not important enough for them to be there for my birthday. Going with Ben took first priority. We would have presents and cake when they got back, but I never had a party with my friends. While they went hunting, I usually had to stay with one of my mom's friends in our neighborhood or my friend's grandmother would come and stay with me at our house. Through all this time, year after year, the underlying thought communicated to me was that Ben always came first and what I wanted or needed was not as important. I was not worth celebrating or having a special day. I finally had a birthday party with my friends, but it was not until my senior year in high school before I went off to college.

Mom and I did not go to church because we had no way to get there. She would turn on the radio and listen to Billy

Graham every Sunday morning and when his Crusades were on television, we would watch them. I learned when I was older that both my mom and dad gave their lives to Christ at a Billy Graham Crusade in the 1950s. They were active in the Youth for Christ ministry. Through the radio programs and crusades, I heard the Word of God and knew what sin was and what would be the penalty. I also knew that Christ had died to save us from those sins and give us eternal life. When I was around nine years old, I believed I accepted Christ, but it was not true repentance. I bargained with God in a cry for help. I told God I would become a Christian if He would stop what was going on with Mom and Ben. Nothing really changed.

When I started junior high, a neighbor down the street, to whom I am eternally grateful, invited me to come to church with her family, and I became part of the youth group there. Through what I learned from God's Word and saw in the lives of the people in the church, I realized that you cannot come to God and bargain. When I was seventeen, while watching a Billy Graham Crusade on television, I knew I had to surrender my life to Christ because I wanted to repent and be forgiven of my sins, not just to have my situation change. On December 1, 1974, I made that choice. Although the situation didn't change, I now had a place of refuge where I could go and talk to God about it and find peace.

When I was younger I did not understand what was really going on with Mom and Ben. But as I got into junior high and high school and heard other kids talk about sex, I began to realize the truth. My mom was really Ben's mistress. Ben paid for everything we had: our house, food, clothes, etc. We did not have a car, so we could only go somewhere when he could take us. I never could go to my friends' houses either, unless I went home with them from school and they brought me back to my house.

When I was in high school I never wanted to have any of my friends come over to my house because I did not know how to introduce or explain Ben to them. I wouldn't say he was my father, but I had learned not to say he was my mom's boyfriend either. I thought if I could figure out what was going on between them, other people could, too. I felt so ashamed and thought people would think I was "bad" like my mom.

As I was in my last two years of high school, Ben began making lewd and suggestive comments to me in front of my mother. She never said a word. I usually ignored it or made an excuse to leave the room. A couple of times he touched me inappropriately, making it seem like he was joking. I told him to stop, that I didn't like to be touched like that. He got very angry and yelled at me, calling me a tease and told me to go to my room. My mom never stepped in or talked to me about it. She just pretended nothing happened. Again, she chose him over me.

As I started dating, I was reluctant to be touched by my date. It took some time before I even felt comfortable holding hands. Between the abuse as a young child and the advances from Ben, I was terrified by the thought of being touched by a male. Slowly, through the relationships I had in high school and college, I realized that not all boys or men were bad or wanted to take advantage of me. But this new perspective of men brought with it a great sadness and grieving, as I realized how much I had wanted and missed the affection a father and daughter share in an appropriate setting.

God has truly blessed me with my wonderful husband, Nick. He knew about my family background before we were married and he told me he would never leave me or mistreat me. Because I was so against my mother's behavior and determined not to be like her, I went to the other extreme and wanted very little to do with sex, even with my husband.

Nick showed extreme patience with me after we married as we worked through my fears of having sex. There aren't too many young men in their early twenties, with all that pent up sexual desire, who would put up with a wife who had no desire for intimacy. I thought of sex as a wife's duty, a distasteful obligation that was forced upon her. There was no pleasure in it for her, just a body to be taken at the whim of a man. I could not see that God created it to be something beautiful between a husband and wife, something that joined them together in body and spirit. Over the years I enjoyed sex better, but I still was not the initiator.

My breakthrough came in 2003 when I went to counseling after my emotional breakdown. My therapist helped me to talk through my feelings about intimacy and gave me books and other resources that helped me discover what God intended marital sex to be. Finally, after twenty-five years of marriage, I was able to desire and enjoy making love with my husband. My only regret was all the years that were wasted not enjoying something so precious. I know our marriage would not have lasted without Nick's patience, support, and encouragement in telling me that I could change the way I viewed intimacy. We have learned together to be open and talk about the area of sex as we have faced the changes that come with aging and menopause. This communication is the key to keeping the closeness and love alive in our marriage and, really, in anyone's marriage.

As for my mom and Ben, my mom moved in with my grandmother for over three years to take care of her because my grandmother was dying of cancer. After her death, my mom returned to find that Ben had married another woman. Since the only income Mom had was her social security, she had to move into subsidized senior housing. A few years after Mom came back, Ben died suddenly. She had given him more than thirty years of her life and she ended up poor and alone, while his new wife got everything he had built over his life.

As you will see later in the book, I struggled to reconcile with my mom on this issue with Ben. She did not want to talk about it, and I left it alone. Some of the dreams paint her in a harsh light, but please remember these are the emotions of a child being expressed as an adult. I don't want you to think I hated my mom. I loved her dearly. I am not responsible for her choices, but I am responsible for how I let those choices impact my life as an adult.

When mom moved into HUD housing after finding out about Ben's marriage, she built herself a brand new life. She started attending the "Hello Club," which consisted of professors' wives who did charitable work. Mom loved catering and hosting elaborate teas for them, complete with decorations, finger sandwiches, and desserts. Eventually, she became a tour guide and took the wives on weekend trips to the big city for shopping and the art museum exhibits. She loved this part of her life. As they rode on the bus to the city, she had games for them to play, with small prizes. The women enjoyed these trips and were always excited to see what she had in mind for the next trip.

Over the last fifteen years my mom lived in an assisted living facility. She carried on her hospitable and caring ways with catered private dinners for her friends and planning day trips to take in the van. She was of great assistance to the chef in what older people like to eat and helped the activities director in planning special events.

In 2016 she fell and hit her head, which caused the onset of severe dementia and forced us to put her into a nursing home. Over the next few months, I drew closer to my mom during our bi-weekly visits and we talked about the old times she could remember.

On Thanksgiving Day in 2017 my mom passed away peacefully. I choose to remember her as the vibrant, caring, fun person she was in the second half of her life, rather than the first half.

# 3

# Beginnings of Depression

As I have said before, I was stunted emotionally most of my life from the age of four until I came to a crisis point in my forties. I put up an emotional wall as a child to block out what had happened to me. As I grew up, my normal coping mechanism for dealing with strong emotions and stressful situations was to keep overly busy so I had no time to think about or deal with the emotions, or I just ignored them and stuffed them down inside. But there came a time when even that strategy could no longer help.

In 1999, I received a call from the doctor saying they saw a suspicious lump on my mammogram and wanted to do further testing. The ultrasound showed a lump and a cyst next to each other. This finding scared me because my mother's mother and sister both had breast cancer and ultimately died from it. Was I going to have it, too? Different scenarios raced through my mind. Also, Nick's mother died from breast cancer, so it was scary for him in a different way. We just held each other and prayed God would help us get through this no matter what the outcome. We let some of our close friends know and we could feel the support of their prayers.

The doctor decided to do a breast biopsy and remove both the cyst and the lump. The lump came back benign. We were so relieved and very thankful for the answer to many prayers.

A month later I experienced severe abdominal pain while driving home from choir practice. I made it home and Nick rushed me to the emergency room. They found nothing to explain the pain, gave me pain pills, and told me to see my doctor the next day. My doctor did further tests and found cysts on both ovaries. He scheduled surgery for the next afternoon, which was Good Friday.

Sometimes humor breaks the strain of tense situations. In my case, Nick and I went to the grocery store before I reported for surgery so I could get food for Easter Sunday. I could not have anything to eat before the surgery, but I was so hungry. In the store there was a lady giving samples of ham. I picked one up and started to put it in my mouth, when Nick grabbed my hand, reminding me I couldn't eat. It smelled so good and I just licked it over and over and then threw it is the trash can by the lady. Her mouth was open and her eyes were wide in surprise as she just stared at me. I quickly walked away, giggling.

When we got to the hospital later that afternoon, the surgeon said he did not know what he would find when he got inside, but he would try to leave me one ovary. When

I came out of surgery, the doctor explained that there were two cysts on the left ovary and one on the right ovary. He was able to remove the cysts and leave the left ovary, but the right ovary and cyst were so entangled and scarred that he had to remove both of them. I came home on Easter Sunday afternoon very thankful that it had not been ovarian cancer, like my mother had suffered when I was in junior high school.

But that was not the end of the medical situations. In 2000, I broke my leg when I slipped on a wet floor while running errands at lunchtime. I saw a coworker as the paramedics were checking my leg. I asked her to run back to work and get my bag with my purse so I would have my identification and insurance card with me at the hospital. They loaded me into the ambulance. The ambulance ride was not at all like it is on television or in the movies. Both EMTs got into the front of the ambulance and left me by myself in the back. We raced through the streets with the lights flashing and siren screaming, bumping over every pothole along the way. When they got to the nurses' desk in the emergency room, I said I needed to call my husband to tell him what happened. He arrived and they put me out with morphine and temporarily set my leg. When I woke up in the dark the next night, I was disoriented, not sure of where I was. Then I saw my leg hoisted up in traction and realized they had done the surgery. They put a rod down the tibia bone and anchored it with screws in my knee and ankle. I missed two months of work and then, while on crutches, I resumed commuting by train to work for six more months before the cast came off. Eighteen months later I had another surgery to remove the rod and screws, with more time off work and more physical therapy.

After the stress of all of these medical problems, several very emotional life events occurred in 2002 over a short period of time, and the culmination of all of these occurrences ultimately sent me over the brink. Within a six-week span, my husband graduated with his doctoral degree, our oldest daughter graduated from college, our youngest daughter graduated from high school, and then our oldest daughter got married. Those things would be enough to challenge even a sane person, let alone one in a fragile mental state. However, in addition to all of those events, two months after the wedding my mother was diagnosed with breast cancer and had a mastectomy. I went to stay with her for a week when she came home from the hospital. Then I went back home and had only three days to shop and pack up our youngest daughter to take her to college for her freshman year.

That autumn I began struggling with the empty nest syndrome, trying to figure out who I was now. In a daily sense, I was no longer a mom. I didn't drive kids anywhere, have conversations with them over dinner, or make sure their homework was finished. It seemed like the phone never rang after they left home. I didn't know what my purpose was now that they were raised and on their own.

Throughout the next year my mom began having a series of mini-strokes, and we decided it would be better to move her into an assisted living facility near my home. In September 2003, we moved her to her new home. Due to the mastectomy, she had edema in her arm and she could not lift anything over five pounds or raise her arm over her head, so I needed to help her unpack and put away her things in her new apartment.

Every day for two weeks, I was gone from home eleven hours for work and commuting, then grabbed something to eat, and went to her place for a couple of hours to unpack what I could. On the weekends my husband and I would go spend a few hours emptying more boxes.

The compounding of these events one on top of the other within a four-year span, especially the last fifteen months, brought all of my coping skills to a halt. I woke up one morning and simply couldn't get out of bed. No matter how much my brain said to get up, my body would not obey. I called in sick to work and stayed in bed sleeping the rest of the day. The next day I was able to go to work, but I had difficulty focusing on tasks and concentrating on my work. By the time I got home, I was exhausted and went straight to bed. I didn't even want to eat dinner.

Several days went on in this fashion, and I talked to my husband about seeking counseling to determine what was going on with me. I found out later that he realized almost a year earlier that I needed professional help, but I was not able to see it yet. This downward spiral was very difficult for him to watch, knowing he could not force me to seek help; I had to come to the realization and want it for myself. It took some time to find a therapist who accepted our insurance and who did not know my husband professionally. I finally found someone and started going to therapy at night. When I recounted the series of events for him, he shook his head and said he was amazed I survived this long before seeing a counselor. I told him I kept putting it off because I was afraid I would break down and start crying, and once I started I would not be able to stop.

Because of shutting off any deep emotions most of my life, I lived mostly on the surface with my feelings. My therapist wanted me to be able to identify what emotions I was experiencing, so he had me write in a journal three emotions I recognized experiencing every day. Even after I got better at identifying the emotions, I kept up the journal to see my progress.

During the initial breakdown period, I had one of my scariest moments. One day I went to the grocery store to pick up a few items, maybe five things on my list. I went up and down the aisles looking at the list and then at the shelves. After half an hour I gave up and went home. When I arrived home Nick asked me where I put the groceries. I sat down on the couch, sobbing. He was really worried and asked again about the groceries. I looked up at him, tears streaming down my face, and choked out the words, "I couldn't find them."

My brain had overloaded with all that was going on and it could not make the connection between what my eyes saw on the list and the items on the shelves. I looked right at the item but could not process in my mind that it was the item I was looking for. That episode made me feel like I really was losing my mind.

When I told my therapist about the episode, he said I needed to stop everything I was involved in and let my brain rest. I could only go to work and to church on Sunday morning. I could not do any of the activities I had been doing at church such as Sunday school or singing in the choir. Interaction with people drained me too much emotionally, and it took all I had just to get through work each day. He said the amount of activities I had been doing was not normal for anyone. Yet almost everyone around me was living the same way, with work and kid's activities each night and struggling to keep up with it all.

He said I needed to find what my "new normal" was going to be from this point forward. I could not go back to that former life and keep my sanity. It was so hard to let go of all the things I had been doing. Like many people, I gauged my self-worth by what I did and what I accomplished. I concerned myself with what people thought of me based on how well my kids or husband looked or acted. Eventually, through a lot of hard work at discovering my boundaries and finding ways to relax, like listening to soothing music or going for a walk, I was able to feel the weight from all of the expectations, both from myself and others, being lifted off my shoulders. I learned how much activity I could handle emotionally and how much would trigger the feeling of being overwhelmed. I began to recognize the symptoms of fatigue and hopelessness coming on and I could take steps, such as journaling my feelings or talking to a friend, and avoid a depressive episode.

For example, a regular week in my previous schedule used to be working all week, sometimes up to 55 hours, going to an event on Friday night, grocery shopping on Saturday morning and visiting my mom or running errands Saturday afternoon, then on Sunday going to church and getting ready for the next week. I realized I had to limit my interaction with other people to only one event other than church on the weekend and reduce my hours at work.

At first, when I thought I needed to take a short nap or rest, I felt guilty because I wasn't doing much around the house and Nick was shouldering a lot of the chores that were normally mine, as well as his own chores. When I had to tell someone that I could not help them with a project or serving in some way, I believed I was letting them down and just being lazy. One of the hardest lessons I learned, but by far the most important and freeing, was that I was of value and worth, and I needed to take care of my own well-being. I had to develop the ability to feel okay about saying no to others. My therapist said that I had to give both my mind and body time to rest and heal. If all I could do when I got home was empty the dishwasher and go to bed, that was okay.

I could tell when I was getting overwhelmed because I had trouble concentrating on things for very long periods of time. I would become obsessive-compulsive in making lists and rehearsing them over and over. While at work, I would make a list of what I needed to do when I got home. It wasn't just a list such as do the dishes, laundry, etc. I made a list of every movement: walk to the train, take the train home, drive home from the train station, come into the house, change clothes, go to the kitchen, fix dinner, eat dinner, go through the mail, put out clothes for tomorrow, wash face, brush teeth, go to bed. I would pull this list out and read it over and over trying to get the steps fixed in my head. I kept rehearsing the list to get the information on the paper to register in my brain because when I didn't look at the paper, I couldn't remember the steps. I also wanted to sleep all the time, like a bear in hibernation. The fatigue, both physical and mental, is pretty typical with depression. Dealing with the emotions robs your energy.

Through this time of readjusting my life, I learned something that has been invaluable to me ever since. I had to give myself permission to do nothing or let something go and not feel guilty about it. It took some time to master, but I realized the price I had to pay for doing too much was not worth the cost to my physical and emotional health. When I thought about doing an activity, I had to stop and ask myself what impact this activity would have on my family and me. Did I have enough rest time prior to the event so I could handle the emotional exertion? Would I need to let something go in order to participate in this activity? I still continue the practice today of asking myself these questions to evaluate whether to be involved in some type of ministry or to participate in an activity. I ask myself if choosing to say yes to the activity will be helpful or harmful to me. For instance, if I am asked if I can make and serve snacks for VBS, I say I will look at my calendar and call them back. If I have nothing scheduled in the evening that week, then I might make snacks one evening and then help serve them at VBS two other nights. But if I have something else on one or two nights, then I will only agree to make snacks one night and not serve at VBS. If people are disappointed or don't understand my answer, I tell myself I cannot control their reactions, but I am at peace inwardly because I know my answer is the best one for me to take care of myself.

I still take naps on weekends, especially in the winter when it is darker, but I am able to say to myself, "You need to do the laundry, but you also need rest. Start the laundry and it will be ready to finish when you get up." I am much better now at knowing when I need to say no to something and get rest, instead of pushing myself to get everything done.

# 4

# Introduction to Dreams

As I progressed through my counseling sessions, I began having dreams so vivid that I could still remember them when I woke up. I wrote them down in my journal and talked about them with my therapist. He had never heard of anyone who had dreams so detailed and realistic, along with the insight into what the dreams were saying or what they meant to me. Going forward in this book, I want to share some of those dreams to demonstrate how God brought healing to my life.

I have arranged the dreams, along with the interpretations that God revealed to me, topically and then chronologically within the topic. My intent is that you will see the different areas in which God was at work in my circumstances and in me during the depression and afterward. It will also allow you to see the progression in the healing process by providing dates of the dreams.

Before I begin describing how God used the dreams to bring healing to my heart, soul, mind, and emotions, I want to tell you about several recurring characters in the dreams. One of them is Scott, my best friend in high school. We could talk about anything with each other, even our relationships with other people we were dating. We even dated briefly but decided we really were better off just being best friends. One of the subjects Scott and I never talked about was Ben. From the times he had been at my house, I believed Scott was aware of my home situation and Ben, but the greatest gift he gave me was that he liked me for who I was and did not judge me because of my mom's lifestyle choices. In my dreams, whenever the subject matter became too hard for me to process or it was too scary for me to face, Scott would come into my dream and I would calm down and not be afraid. Because he had accepted me unconditionally, he was where I felt safe and protected. You will also see my husband playing this role of safety at times in the dreams.

One of the other recurring themes is the location, specifically two distinct places. First, in several dreams I am at a church or there is a reference to a church. I was struggling with my relationship with God and whether I could trust Him to be in control of my life. I believe the references to churches helped me see that God was always there with me, whether I could see it or not. He never left me and He was wooing me back to Himself. I was learning that rather than the church itself, God was the real source of my help and healing, although sometimes it came through the body of believers.

The other place is a school or classroom setting. I believe it symbolized the learning I had to do to see the truth of who I was and who God was, how to let go of things that were hindering my life, and how to be healthy physically, mentally, and spiritually.

Many of the dreams are about anger towards my mom and Ben and deal with sexual issues, but I believe some of those dreams are not about them. The dreams use Mom and Ben as familiar objects to direct my feelings regarding the molestation. I never felt a lot of hostility earlier in my life about this, but I think some of the situations with Mom and Ben brought out the reactions I couldn't express as a child about the molestation. With better understanding as an adult, I now could put words and feelings to that situation and to the incidents with Mom and Ben.

The final character seen over and over in my dreams is some type of child. Sometimes it is clearly a boy or a girl; other times it is just a generic toddler or child. In some instances, the child is by itself and I am trying to protect it from others. On other occasions, the child is traveling with me and we are going through situations together. In some of the dreams I am the character, but it feels like I am watching the events from outside of the dream. My therapist said the child was a representation of me. In order to cope with what was happening to me from ages three to five, I retreated emotionally and spent the next forty years stuck in that childlike level. He affirmed that I have been a good mom to my children and encouraged me to be a mom to this child to help my emotions grow beyond the place where they had stagnated. My hope is that you will be able to see the changes in the child as the dreams progress through time.

# 5

# Dreams Dealing with Anger, Guilt, and Shame

## May 17, 2004—Treatment by Others

Nick came home and said we were moving. He had sold the house and found an apartment for us. I got really angry that he would do something like that without talking to me about it first. I told him I was not going to live in an apartment because I wanted a yard and space. I did not want neighbors hearing everything we did. He said he didn't want to have to do yard work and take care of a house. There was a lot of yelling back and forth.

The scene changed and I was walking down the aisle of a bus looking for someplace to sit. I was very tired. I made my way to the back of the bus but it looked more like the back of a station wagon. Working my way to the rear,

I realized the person in the corner was Scott. I snuggled in next to him and went to sleep. When I woke up we weren't in the bus anymore. We were walking along a sidewalk through a neighborhood, catching up with each other on what was happening in our lives. I felt safe, secure, and happy. When we reached the next corner, I said goodbye and walked further down the street as he turned at the corner and walked away.

## Interpretation

The dream was not really about Nick and me arguing or his making decisions without me. It was about people telling me how to "get over" my depression. I felt as though I didn't have a voice in my own treatment.

Now I was standing up for myself and acknowledging my need for help. My focus was on trying to take charge of my own recovery through seeing a therapist and finding ways to restrict my participation in things that would intensify the depression. During the chaos represented by the arguing, Scott was there representing someone who was safe and secure, someone who would listen and understand. Some people didn't understand how I could say no to helping with cleanup day at church or helping at the soup kitchen because they see being constantly busy as a normal life, as I did before, so I seem abnormal. Perhaps deep down they want to slow down and be okay with saying no sometimes, but going against the current culture is too frightening.

When I make a stand about my choice to be less busy or I have emotional interactions with others that tax my emotions, I still get scared about my depression and run back to where I feel safe. I am learning that I need to run to God. He is always holding me securely in His hands.

## August 19, 2004—Feeling Left Out

When I first came into the sanctuary of a church, I saw Nick but ignored him because I was furious with him. He was the reason we moved to this new place and I just sat in the nearest pew with a scowl on my face. When he tried to talk to me, I told him to leave me alone.

As the service began, I looked at the platform and noticed a friend of mine was leading the music. After the service, I asked my friend if I could help with the music even though this wasn't my church. I felt jealous of her singing, but at the same time felt left out because no one ever asked me to help sing or lead music.

The scene changed and Nick and I were in a different church service and we were sitting together, but I still felt distant from him. In the middle of the service I went to a small room just off of the sanctuary. Nick and a couple of our friends followed me. They tried to talk to me, but I just ignored them and refused to talk. They wanted to know what was wrong, but I just got more upset and kept quiet. One of my friends kept pushing me to say why I was acting this way. That's when I snapped. I hit a table really hard with my fist (in reality I jerked my leg and hit the dog on our bed). I screamed at them that I hated God, I hated my life, and I was tired of being everyone's charity case. I didn't like people giving us food and looking at me with that "poor thing" attitude. I hated not being able to buy things. All of my friends talked about what they were doing at church or in the community and I couldn't join in the conversation because I was so inactive. My depression kept me from singing or helping at church or going out for fun with my friends. I had no life outside of my job. I sat down, sobbing into my hands.

## Interpretation

I was angry about the way my life was at the time. I felt as if every day was always the same. Nothing in my daily routine ever changed. I went to work at 7:00 a.m. and came home around 6:00 p.m., but some nights it was after 10:00 p.m., then I got up the next morning and did it all over again. Weekends were spent running errands and taking care of the house and my family. I worked about fifty hours a week to pay for everyone in the family to go to college. What about my dreams and ambitions? I wanted to work with animals, but we couldn't afford for me to quit work and go to school. When did I get to do something for me? How long would my life continue without any fun or excitement?

I knew in my mind that working so much was temporary until my husband and both children were done with college, but that would take several years. Emotionally and physically I was exhausted and blamed everyone else for my unhappiness with life. Later, when we moved away after everyone finished college, I was able to get a job at a veterinary office. Nick was very supportive of me pursuing my dream and taking classes to be a veterinary assistant. It was finally my turn.

## September 26, 2004—Wanting to Be Understood

My friend, Jan, was hosting a surprise fortieth birthday party for our mutual friend, Susan, and I was helping her get things ready. I asked Jan where she wanted the other helpers to set up the tables and chairs. Although we were all busy decorating and making food, I was happy working with others. When Susan came into the room, everyone yelled, "Surprise!" while clapping and cheering. After the dinner, Jan showed a video depicting various times in Susan's life.

I noticed my mom was at the party. The narrator of the video referred to Susan's husband, who was in the doctoral program with my husband. Mom asked the man next to her if I was going to be in this part and he nodded yes. The narrator then began talking about my story—the abuse when I lived with my dad and the living situation with Mom and Ben. Mom said sarcastically, "Oh yeah, that was really hard for her." But she was so loud that no one could hear what the narrator was saying. I wanted to tell her to be quiet because no one could hear over her voice. However, all I could do was get up and leave.

I went into the library that had bookshelves lining two walls and inhaled the comforting smell of leather and books. I sat down in one of the big leather chairs and cried. Nick came in to see if I was okay. I was furious at Mom and said, "Why does she have to do this in front of everyone?

She acts so self-righteous, but she doesn't even hear what I am saying to her."

I got up and went downstairs to see if I could help clean up the dishes from dinner. I did not realize I was dressed in only my bra and panties. I passed through the room where everyone had been gathered, thinking the program must be finished by now, but Mom was still ranting. I was so embarrassed. I went back to the library and curled up on the leather couch. Mom came looking for me. I told her that she didn't belong here and that she needed to go home and leave me alone.

## Interpretation

I was having some success at being comfortable around other people and I felt better with my depression. I could interact a little with others and be helpful to some extent, but it was too overwhelming to be in charge of anything. I wanted to share my story with others about the work God was doing in me. I was angry with Mom. Our relationship was strained because it seemed as if she was keeping everyone from hearing my story and the feelings I was trying to express. She wasn't actually doing anything; instead, I was harboring anger towards her and it was getting in the way.

Nick coming to see if I was okay represents a protector, someone who was encouraging me and taking care of me.

The reference to being in my bra and panties shows how vulnerable I was feeling when I shared with others. I was putting myself out there where I could be rejected, and when I tried to share with Mom, she did not want to hear it. She just tried to justify her actions to me.

## November 7, 2004—Shame by Association

The dream opened at a party in a college dorm. Several people sat on couches, talking and playing board games. Nick was in the kitchen getting some food. A good friend of mine was there, but when I first saw him I couldn't think of his name. I walked over to him, and we chatted about what was going on in our jobs. As we talked, he was slowly and gently rubbing my chest. We moved on separately to mingle and chat with other people, but from time to time we would make eye contact and smile. When it started getting late, people left the party and went home.

The scene changed, and I was at what seemed to be a dinner or banquet with tables scattered around the room, covered with white tablecloths and beautiful centerpieces of yellow roses. I recognized a couple of people from church at one table and my mom was with them, so I joined them. Before the dinner commenced, a man got up to welcome everyone and pray for the meal. After the prayer he said that there were two people in the room who were guilty of fornication and before the evening was over they should come forward to confess and repent. I could hear Mom whisper something to my friends and mentioning my name, but I could not make out what she said, other than, "from top to bottom." I was so embarrassed, mortified, and angry, but I felt frozen in place, unable to speak. I moved to another table and ignored her the rest of the evening.

When I went to get food from the buffet line, everyone was looking at me and whispering. I heard someone say all I needed was a scarlet letter. I kept moving back and forth around the room, pretending to get different food so I would not have to sit back down. Nick arrived late to the dinner after all of this had happened. I told him what happened and he stood by me, telling me not to pay attention to what they said because I knew it wasn't true. I told him I wanted to go home. I was so deeply embarrassed and humiliated that I couldn't face these people any longer.

## Interpretation

My friend's inappropriate touching represented the temptation and lure for me to become promiscuous like Mom. Mom's comments about me to my friends at the table pointed to Mom's hypocrisy in real life. She might say negative things about my life but was oblivious to her own shortcomings. She would rant about the immorality of young people in the 1960s and 1970s, but she would never admit to her own adultery.

Research shows that quite often children who have been sexually abused end up in prostitution because of their low self-esteem, because it is what they know how to do, and/or because they want someone to care about them. Sometimes they also become abusers themselves because they think such behavior is normal. It is the only model they have witnessed. I thank God He protected me from those paths, even though I couldn't see His working on my behalf at the time.

The reference to the scarlet letter for adultery was how I thought other people looked at me as my mom's daughter and the guilt and shame associated with that perception. I didn't respond to Mom in the dream because I didn't know what she had said. In real life, I couldn't stand up for myself and tell her how I felt embarrassed by her lifestyle and what people would say about us. When I was young I didn't want to have friends over to my house because they might discover how I lived and think I was immoral like my mom. I felt dirty and unworthy of having friends.

I loved the part about Nick standing up for me because it expressed how he affirmed me during therapy and my working through these emotions. He told me the truth, I was not a slut or whore, I was not like my mom, and there was no reason to feel guilty or ashamed.

The scene about being in school represented how God was still teaching me the truth about myself. He was showing me that the sexual abuse when I lived with my dad and the consequences of Mom's choices were not my fault and they did not have to dictate how I saw myself or define who I could become. I did not have to follow those paths. I could choose to be something better and follow the path God had planned for me, as I began to see myself as He sees me, pure and cleansed.

## January 28, 2005—Harboring Unforgiveness

I came home from work and started making pork chops and salad for dinner. After dinner, Mom was cleaning off the table and putting the dishes in the sink for me to wash.

She told me I was doing the dishes the wrong way. I should do the cups, then the silverware, then the plates. I didn't bite at her criticism this time. I went into the living room to watch television and left her to do the dishes.

The next morning Mom complained how dusty the dining room was and I lost it and screamed at her, saying, "I'm not the stay-at-home mom like you were, the one who had everything looking like a magazine cover. I don't care if the pillows on the couch are arranged just so or if the dog's food is outside the dish. He'll eat it off the floor."

I was late getting up and getting ready for work. I grabbed my shoes and hurried out the door to the car. Nick said he would drive me to the train station. When I got in the car, Mom was there also. I didn't want her there, but there wasn't time to argue with her, so we drove to the station. When we got there, I was late and had missed my train. I was irritated because now I had to walk to the train station in the next town. They both walked with me and we got there just as the train was pulling into the station. I was still very upset with Mom because now I was going to be late for work. I apologized to Nick for snapping at him when I got out of the car. I knew it wasn't his fault we were late.

As I got off the train at the downtown station, Mom got off with me. I got on the bus that went close to my office and so did Mom. I refused to talk to her. She started to get off at the same stop with me, but I stopped her and asked where she was going. She didn't answer me. I was angry that she was following me everywhere.

The scene changed and I was at my friend Katy's house and several of us were going to drive to school together. Katy was very slow getting ready. I got impatient with her and told her to hurry up. It was 9:00 in the morning and I asked what time school started. Katy said it started at 7:15 a.m. I yelled, "Let's go. We've already missed two classes!"

I went out on the porch and realized I had forgotten my backpack so I ran back inside to get it. When I came back to the car, Mom was sitting in the driver's seat. As I got in, she started pulling down the driveway. I told her to stop so Katy and the others wouldn't have to walk so far. She was insolent, but she stopped and everyone got into the car. We got to school really late and I found myself wandering around the hallways alone.

The school looked scary. It had dirty, unfinished cinderblock walls and the bathroom had no door, so you could see people standing at the urinals. Students were huddled in the hallway, but no one made a sound. They just stared at me with vacant looks on their faces. I found my way to the office and the principal said he would show me the orientation film and then I could go to class. I ended up sitting next to a girl who was an obnoxious chain smoker. When the film was over, all of the students left to pick up class schedules and get to class. I was all alone again, standing at the bottom of a set of stairs so high that I could not see the top of them. I had to climb these stairs to get to my class.

## Interpretation

I didn't want to think about my attitude toward Mom. I wanted to keep my distance from her, even though I went to see her once a week, because I was not ready to confront her emotionally in a healthy way. I was afraid I would get so mad that I would yell at her like I did in the dream, and it would harm our relationship for the future. I resented having to take care of Mom now in her later life, even though she did not take care of me when I was little.

However, I could see a little growth and healing in my attitude and emotions because there was a part of me that wanted to reconcile with her. I just was not yet able to talk to her in a calm and respectful manner about how I felt. No matter what she had done, she was still my mom and I needed to honor her.

The school represented God teaching me who He wants me to be and to come to a place where I can forgive Mom, letting go of the anger. The school looking bleak and uncomfortable with urinals out in the open represented how scared and exposed I felt about sharing my feelings with Mom. Learning how to deal with my depression was hard because I had to confront things that were hurtful and sad both in her and in me. I thought I had to tackle my lack of forgiveness toward Mom by myself. But God was teaching me that I could not do it in my own strength. Only He could heal the hurt and anger I felt. He promised that He would be faithful to heal me if I would give my inability to forgive over to Him.

Missing the train and having Mom follow me represented carrying the anger with me everywhere I went, even into other relationships. My bitterness was controlling me, and I was damaging my relationships with my family and friends.

The outburst about cleaning the house was about my vexation with Mom when she would criticize how I was living my life. She did not understand, since she stayed at home when I was growing up. She didn't know what it was like to work full-time away from home and then come home to a family and still have to cook supper, clean the house, do the laundry, raise two kids, grocery shop on the weekends, or all the other things that happen in everyday life. I thought her criticism was unfair.

The school also mirrored my life at that point in time: being afraid of moving into a new career, not knowing if I would be good at it, being afraid of failing. The long stairs were a picture of the steep, upward climb in the process of healing, yet I could not see any end.

## May 8, 2005—Standing Up for Myself

As the dream began, I was not a young child, but somewhat older. I walked up on the porch of the house where I grew up and the front door was unlocked. I saw Mom in the kitchen when I came in and said hi, then went to my room to put up my books and change clothes. On the way to my room I passed Mom's room, and Ben was standing there with his underwear partly on. I didn't know if they had just finished having sex or if he was getting ready to and was waiting for Mom. He was fumbling, trying to hurry and get dressed. I said to him, "Again? Don't you ever quit? You are pathetic." He told me to go to my room. He was not yelling, more passive, almost as if he were embarrassed and afraid of me.

When I had first come into the house, Mom said there was an article she left for me on my desk. The article was about parents not being honest with their children and the impact it has on the child's life. I saw the article as her attempt to apologize for the lies she had told me.

Ben came out of the room fully dressed and sheepishly tried to be mad at me, but I told him, "Save your breath. I am tired of you flaunting your adultery in my face. I have homework to do and I don't have time for your foolishness," and shut my door in his face. I was in charge! Neither of them could be mad at me. My life was on my terms, not theirs. I would not quiver in the shadows any longer.

## Interpretation

While I could never have said the things I said in the dream when I was young, the house being unlocked was a symbol of my freedom from being shut out by them as I had been as a child. I was standing up to them and no longer felt humiliated by them. I would not let myself be under their control.

Mocking and ridiculing them made me feel in charge of my own life because I could speak the truth to them and live in that freedom. They were timid and afraid of me because I would not cower before them and meekly do what they said. I now had the power, through God's Word and the love He showed me, to say that I choose to live my life without the fear and shame from my past.

## October 12, 2005—Loss of My Father

In my dream, I received a phone call from Mom saying she and Ben were leaving that afternoon and would arrive at my house the next day, but I wasn't really listening to her. At work the next day, the receptionist said I had a call and that it was my father. I thought, "This should be interesting," so I took the call. It was Ben and he said he was coming to see me that afternoon. I was furious! When he showed up I took him into a conference room and closed the door. I yelled, "How dare you tell people you are my father!" and told him to leave. He said that he and Mom would be back next Thursday, and I needed to pick them up at the airport at 4:00 p.m. I sarcastically asked where they were going this time, and he said they were going to Hawaii. I told him I was sorry, but he had to leave the building. I needed to hurry or I would miss my train. He said he would drive me to the station. I answered, "No thanks. I would rather miss my train than ride with you."

## Interpretation

I was so angry with Ben because I didn't want him to think he could replace my father, to assume that role. Most people who encountered the three of us together would assume that he was my father by the way he acted. To my child's mind, he was just as bad as my father. It seemed at

40

times that Ben didn't really want me around; I just came in the package with Mom. I didn't have the legitimacy or place of belonging that his kids had. I know as I look back as an adult that he did actually care about me like one of his own, but still I was always the third wheel. I realized his children actually had it worse than me because he was hardly ever home. They did not have much time with him at all when they were growing up.

Picking Mom and Ben up at the airport represented the demands I was feeling taking care of Mom. On top of everything else I was responsible for, I was her taxi service, chewing up even more of my Saturdays doing things for her. I know this sounds very selfish and a mean way to speak about my mom. Of course, I would do anything to help her because she was my mother and I loved her. But in the grip of depression, I felt completely overwhelmed by all the responsibilities on my plate. I realized I had to start making boundaries with Mom in order to take care of myself. Sometimes I needed to tell her no, I couldn't be there Saturday, without feeling guilty about it and see if I could offer an alternate time when I could come.

My anger at their trip to Hawaii was a picture of my resentment that they were going away without me, as they did when I was little. I didn't belong with them; I was just in the way of what they wanted to do. I was to stay home with strangers and behave, but I wasn't welcome to go along on vacations.

## March 10, 2011—Resentment for Lifestyle

Mom, Ben, and I, as an adult, got out of the car and went into our backyard. I looked over to my right and noticed a big vehicle in our backyard. It was the size of a bus, but it was shaped differently. I went over to look at it and saw it had a tarp across the back where you could reach inside. Ben said it was the trailer they used to transport the horses to his horse competitions. I got excited that there might be horses inside. I opened the tarp and there were six horses in the trailer. I reached inside and patted a beautiful gray horse with a long black mane, talking to it gently.

I heard Ben tell Mom that he was cleaning out the barn so he had to get all the horses out. He said they were redoing the stalls for his horses. I stopped patting the horse, closed the tarp and stomped off towards the house. Mom asked what was wrong with me, and I said, "Oh sure, you get whatever you want and I get squat!" I went into the house, slamming the door and locking it. Then I went to my room and locked that door.

Mom and Ben were pounding on the door to the house, yelling at me to let them in, but I just ignored them. Ben took out his keys and unlocked the door then came and started banging on my bedroom door, telling me to open it. I said no. I asked, "How does it feel to be locked out of the house and humiliated in front of the neighbors?" They asked me what I meant about not getting squat. What did I want that I did not have? I said I wanted freedom: "Freedom to have a car and go when and where I wanted, to be able to go places with my friends, to have my own money to spend, not what was doled out to us by Ben. I did not ask to be part of this living arrangement; I just got stuck in it. I wanted to leave and go live with my aunt and uncle and have a normal life."

## Interpretation

The dream was about my resentment at having to hear all about his horses and the competitions he won. I loved horses and desperately wanted one, but I could not have one in a neighborhood subdivision. He had the life I thought I wanted.

I also was expressing my frustration for being kept like Mom, having everything given to us by Ben. He bought our house, our food, our clothes, took us wherever we needed to go. I was not able to go to my friends' houses or activities after school because his schedule did not allow him to take me or pick me up. Mom never saw any of my track meets and only a couple of my choral concerts in high school. I was angry that I was stuck in this situation because of Mom, and I just wanted to go and live a regular life like other people lived.

Locking them out was an attempt to shut them out of my life. I didn't want them deciding what I could do or where I could go. Yelling at them about what I wanted and what I was missing was my way of getting them to see how life was from my point of view. I wanted them to understand that I felt isolated and alone.

I had kept the emotions relating to how I felt about Ben's family and what our living situation took away from me bottled up as a child, because if I ever expressed these feelings out loud to either of them I would have been punished. God brought the anger and bitterness I was feeling to the surface through my dream, where my subconscious could express the hurt and frustration out loud as I had always wanted to do when I was younger.

As I read the dream over later, the anger and resentment no longer felt as deep or visceral as it did before. Thinking about the things I wanted but couldn't have and things I missed out on helped me, over time, to see and grieve the losses from the proper perspective. God sees the whole plan, not just a little piece like we do. There is a reason for everything that happens in our lives. The anger and resentment connected to my memories of those events no longer had the same power or control over me. The memories just made me sad.

## May 9, 2011—Wanting Reconciliation

In my dream I went to Mom's house. She invited me in and asked if I wanted some lunch. I told her thanks, but I didn't have time. I had something I wanted to discuss with her. I just wanted her to understand how her relationship with Ben affected me when I was growing up.

When I tried to talk to her about it on other occasions, she just dismissed it, made light of it, or refused to talk about it. I told her sometimes her silence made me so angry I wanted to pinch, punch, or physically hurt her. The pain was so unbearable that I wanted to lash out and punish her. I came to talk to her because I didn't want to be angry with her anymore or have these violent thoughts. I asked her if she would please help me get over these emotions by talking with me about how my childhood looked from my perspective. She wouldn't answer me, so I got up and left.

Later I saw her with a couple of ladies at a coffee shop and I overheard her telling them what I said to her earlier. I came up to their table and shouted at her to talk to me, not to other people. How can she talk to them about this situation but clam up when I want to talk to her? The ladies took up for her, saying I shouldn't speak to her like that. Since she wouldn't even look at me, I left the coffee shop.

That evening as I drove home from work, I came across Mom walking along the side the road. I pulled the car up alongside of her and asked if she wanted me to take her home. She looked at me through the open window of the car, then took off running across a field. I got out of the car and started chasing her, but then I woke up.

## Interpretation

I had attempted to talk to Mom about how I felt. She would never respond to me, other than to say that she never thought about it from my perspective and that she would not apologize for the love they had. I was seeking understanding from her of how it impacted me and to reconcile our relationship, but she refused. I realized this was something she and I would never be able to talk about and I would have to move forward in our relationship without this being resolved between us.

God led me to a point where I could let it go and forgive her. I wrote a letter telling her exactly how I felt and how things from my childhood made me feel, both then and now. I never gave her the letter, but writing it out helped me release the deep hurt and bitterness in my heart and be able to forgive her. We had become close in her later years, but an area in our relationship was closed off. We just talked about the ordinary stuff in our daily lives.

## December 5, 2012—Secret Fear and Shame

I was at a rehearsal for my youth choir concert. Some of the girls who were rich and snobby were picking on me and making fun of me. It was time for me to go onstage to introduce the next song. The girls had changed the stage and props behind my back, so when I walked onstage, it was all wrong and the director yelled at me for not having the stage prepared correctly, while the girls snickered backstage. The director told me to get off the stage and moved on to the next song in the concert.

Backstage I was carrying this tiny box that had a single blue pill in it, but everyone believed the pill was actually a baby. I told them I had a sister, Tilla, who had died. My mom had another baby after Tilla, and this was the new baby. The baby was sick and I had to hold the box at all times to protect it. I had it onstage with me and everyone was very sympathetic and supportive. The story spread and a famous television producer came to our town to do a show about the baby. Just before the show was to start, I opened the box and discovered there were many blue pills instead of just one. I tried taking them out and putting them in my pocket without anyone noticing but I couldn't pick them up out of the box. I didn't want anyone to know the truth that there was no baby. One of the girls from the concert confronted me about the box and I had to admit that it was not really a baby. I apologized to the producer and said I was very sorry for deceiving him and wasting his time. I just missed my sister so much that I made it up. He said it was okay and he would still do the show but from a different angle, talking about how the loss of a sibling affects the family. When I opened the box it was not full of little blue pills, but instead I found many beautiful blue butterflies that fluttered away in the wind.

## Interpretation

I was full of shame about Mom's living situation. I didn't want my friends to come to my house because I was afraid they would learn my secret. I tried to keep the secret close to me, but I lived in constant fear of someone finding out the truth. I would tell lies so they would not figure it out.

The sister dying was a picture of me, my childhood innocence that died when I was molested as a toddler. I didn't want to carry all this grown-up knowledge around with me. I just wanted to have a regular childhood full of playing and being with friends.

The producer in the dream is God. He took the shame and guilt I carried around as a secret and turned it into something stunningly beautiful. But just as there are stages to go through from caterpillar to pupa to butterfly, I saw that God's healing was a process. It was very painful going through the process, and, at times, it seemed as if nothing was happening in that cocoon of waiting. It required me to be patient and trust God, to believe the truth of who He said I was. I had to work hard at changing my mind-set and evaluating my activities to keep me physically and emotionally in balance. I know now that the outcome of transformation in my mind and emotions was worth everything I had to endure on the journey to wholeness. God does make beauty out of ashes! He set me free from the heavy weight of shame. I received the truth that I was beautiful and precious in His eyes.

# 6

# Dreams about
# Sexual Predators

## March 20, 2004—Standing Up
## for a Healthy View of Sex

This dream dealt with healthy sex the way I wanted it to be with my husband. It also was about facing and standing up to the real and figurative predators in my past.

Waking up in the middle of the night and feeling amorous, I started rubbing Nick's chest. He woke up and we began to be intimate. I noticed a light on in the hallway and got out of bed to investigate. Opening the door I screamed in a loud voice, "No, GO AWAY." I came back to bed and started being intimate again. The same thing happened two more times.

I realized that the door in my dream was the same as the door to my room when I was a child, not the door to our room in real life now. When screaming, I had the impression it was Mom and Ben, even though I never saw anyone. I thought they were trying to come in and stop me from making love with my husband, and I was not going to let them.

## Interpretation

I was beginning to believe that sex was not wrong or dirty. It was a good gift from God to be enjoyed between a husband and wife. I was slowly letting go of the shame as a victim of abuse, as if it were my fault or that I was damaged goods. The abuse was a deeply buried secret that I kept from everyone because of the fear of being perceived as immoral or judged by others.

The positive part of the dream was that I stood up to whoever was in the hallway forbidding them from stopping my enjoyment of intimacy with my husband. I would not continue to live under the lie that sex was merely a wife's duty or a lifestyle of an immoral woman. Feeling comfortable with intimacy in the dream was a picture of the kind of intimacy I wanted to have with my husband, even though I wasn't able to feel that freedom yet emotionally. It was the goal worth fighting for with all my heart.

## August 11, 2004—Pursued by Predators

This dream began in a living room. I was lying on a couch on my stomach with my shirt off and Mom was giving me a back rub. Ben entered the room as Mom went to answer the phone. He asked what was going on and I replied, "Mom was giving me a back rub." He said he would finish it and then said, "If I were a good waiter I'd be serving you like this," and he sat me up and kissed me. When Mom came back in, I grabbed my shirt and left the room. I could hear Ben and Mom having a fight about what he was doing to me when she entered the room. He told Mom he would do as he pleased. She gave no response.

The scene changed and as an adult I came into the bedroom and took my clothes off, crawling under the blanket next to Nick. He said he liked the closeness and began fondling my breasts gently. I felt secure and comfortable, with no fear. This experience was so different from what I felt in the previous scene with Ben.

The dream switched back to a scene with Ben. Someone was using a vibrator on me and asked if I was ready yet. Before I could answer or ask what was going on, Ben said that he wanted to be alone with his wife and the other person left. It was like watching the scene from the outside, being removed from what was happening. I could see a man and woman having intercourse, but not clearly see their faces. I had the sense, though, that it was me and Ben.

Then, some teenage girls came into the room when I was dressing. I grabbed up my clothes and went into the bathroom, trying to hide from them. Ben came into the bathroom and asked what I was doing, but I would not come out until the girls left. As the girls departed, they made lewd comments to him about what he was getting and laughed at me.

Suddenly that scene faded away and I was driving a car with a teenage girl in the passenger seat. It was very dark late at night and I was having trouble seeing the road. Everything looked blurry. The girl asked if I knew where we were going. I told her Ben gave me directions to turn left at the third traffic light and then turn left again at the next intersection.

Then everything disappeared. I was standing in a dark hallway and the girl was gone. A woman handed me clothes and told me to get ready, putting me with another girl and told to practice. I was at a strip club, but instead of the women stripping, there were two girls performing various sexual positions with each other.

The scene changed back to the same living room I was in at the beginning of the dream and Ben was finished having intercourse with me. I don't see his face but my mind senses it is him. Mom is lying on a couch nearby with a vacant, death-like stare and not saying a word. I looked around the room and saw my daughter lying on the floor waiting for a back rub. I thought in horror, "She will be next!" Then I woke up breathing hard and shaking all over.

## Interpretation

Ben's comment that he would do as he pleased related to my anxiety that he would molest me. Although he never did molest me, the lewd comments he made to me kept me in constant fear that it might happen.

In contrast, the scene with Nick showed I was believing that good, healthy intimacy was possible for me. I felt comfortable about being touched, rather than being afraid of him. I could trust that he would not harm me.

The teenage girls making vulgar comments and laughing at me, causing me to run out of the room, represented the embarrassment and shame both from the molestation at a young age and living in a home that seemed abnormal from the homes of my friends. I thought people saw me as a slut, an immoral girl, "like mother, like daughter." I couldn't change Mom's lifestyle but could hide the situation by not having my friends come to my house.

The inability to see faces during times of intercourse in the dream illustrates disengaging myself from reality during the molestations when I was young. I assume, from research I've read, that my mind, even though I was small, went to a different place that helped me not be present in what was happening. This avoidance or detachment of the thought process fleeing from reality and going to a familiar or safe place has been shown in various studies to occur often in instances of rape or incest. The mind tries to protect itself from trauma connected to the terrible situation.

Ben gave me the directions to a place that led me to harm. The strippers exposing very private areas and engaging in depraved actions represented the perversions I was exposed to, the stripped bare vulnerability I felt and the lack of protection from those who were supposed to be protecting me.

Mom sitting with a vacant look on her face in the midst of the encounter with Ben and me pictured how she would look the other way and pretend she didn't hear when Ben made lewd comments or passes at me. The daughter in the dream waiting for a back rub was not really my daughter, but she represented the other victims of sexual abuse and incest everywhere. She was the next one in the continual line of abuse. The cycle continues.

## October 30, 2004—Trying to Put the Past behind Me

As the dream commenced, I was at my current house as an adult. It was dark and I was sleeping in my bedroom, and Mom and Ben were in the guest room across the hall. Ben was telling Mom very loudly what to do to him sexually. I got up and went to the door of their room and found it was not quite shut. I burst through the door and angrily asked, "Is it necessary for you to be so loud while having sex, because other people in the house are trying to sleep." He quickly got off the bed and hid on the floor to hide his nakedness.

I knew he would be furious with me for barging into the room and yelling at him. I hurriedly got dressed, grabbed my purse and keys and went outside to the car. I drove for hours until I came to a place that was warm and near a beach and the ocean. It was a place so different from where I had been and it seemed like a good place to stay and find a job.

One day I was walking along the beach feeling the warm sand turn cool as my toes dug beneath the surface. A road ran next to the beach and it was teeming with the traffic of early morning beachgoers. I didn't know Mom and Ben had been looking for me since I left many months ago. I saw a car drive by that had two people in the front seat. It was the same make and model as Ben's car. They did not see me. I realized then how much I had changed in appearance over the last few months. My hair was longer and lighter in color from being in the sun. I had lost a little weight from my daily walks on the beach. Turning around to see where they went, I saw their car stopped in the parking lot next to the marina.

That is when Ben spotted me. He got out of the car and started running toward me, screaming obscenities. I ran to my car parked at a little convenient store and got in. When Ben got close to my car, I backed up out of the parking space, drove in his direction, knocked him down with my car and then drove over him. I backed up and drove over him again and sped away.

## Interpretation

Bursting into the bedroom of Mom and Ben and yelling at Ben illustrated how I was taking control and standing up to them, which I wasn't able to do as a child. Now I was declaring that those memories would not control my life today.

The running away to a beach area somewhat mirrored my real life. I went to college, got married, and moved to Florida, far away from my mom. But the perception that sex was something dirty, something to fear and endure, never went away; it was always lurking in the back of my mind. The things I heard from their room as a child also severely affected the way I made love with my husband because I concentrated so hard on not making any noise instead of enjoying it. I was terrified our children would hear us and be afraid, as I was as a child.

Repeatedly running over Ben with the car symbolized not really killing him, but putting an end to the fear of him molesting me. I was not going to let any kind of fear or shame control my intimacy with my husband any longer.

## February 9, 2011—Preying on the Innocent

I was in the living room playing a board game with a little girl who was about eight years old and her mom was on the couch watching television. The television program showed a naked man holding a big doll in front of his genitals. I ran and turned off the television and started screaming at the woman, "What is wrong with you? How could you have that on in front of a child?" She just sat there staring, oblivious, not uttering a word. I stomped off to my room, yelling all the way there.

But when I got to my room I became afraid for the little girl, so I went back to get her. The mom was still on the couch, but what had been on television was now real. There was the same naked man standing in the doorway to the other bedroom, asking the little girl if she wanted to come play with the doll. The girl started to back away, but the mom said it was okay to go with him.

I could not move. I stood there frozen in place with fear and when I opened my mouth to call the girl, no sound came out. I could not grab the girl fast enough before the man took her into the room. I shouted at the woman to stop the girl, but she just looked at me and said, "It is okay. They are just playing a game." I went and called the police. Before the authorities arrived, I entered the bedroom to get the girl. The woman was now in the bed, but the man and the girl were gone. I asked the woman what happened to them, but she just said everything was all right and refused to say anything else.

The scene changed and the man and woman were chasing me through a field. They were very angry that I had called the police for help and they threatened to get even with me. I woke up before they reached me and never knew what happened to the girl. My heart was pounding and I was gasping for breath.

## Interpretation

The man and woman did not look like Mom and Ben, but the dream made me think about Ben making passes at me and Mom acting nonchalant about it. The part of the dream where I took charge and called for help encouraged me that I was making progress in letting go of the fear and anger. I did not have the same helpless feeling I had as a child. Being able to say now what I wanted to say back then began to release the resentment and bitterness I had carried all those years. I grew up thinking I was not even of enough value to be protected from harm, but now I knew I was of great worth to God and those in my life close to me.

Calling the police was a picture of my cry for help when I had threatened suicide in the note to Mom. I wanted someone to talk to me, to help me understand what was going on with Mom and Ben, and to be assured that Mom was not being injured. Mom just made light of it and told me she did not want to hear any more foolishness about it. She did not try to explain what was happening or allay my fears. She just brushed me aside, pretending everything was okay, like the woman on the couch in the dream, when clearly the child was in danger. One of the hardest areas for me to give over to God and let go of was the anger toward my mom in her passivity to the danger I faced from Ben.

## March 14, 2011—Rescuing the Victims

Walking in the neighborhood, I heard the sound of someone crying coming from the house in front of me. As I approached the house, the woman on the porch said her daughter had been kidnapped. Looking out to the road there was a big moving truck with its back door being shut. There were approximately twenty girls sitting in the truck with their arms around their knees. Once the door was shut, the truck pulled away.

The woman on the porch told me some men were going around to all the towns and taking the girls away. I went to the house two doors down the block and the woman there had hidden her two daughters. I told her I would take the girls to a place that was safe. When leaving, we saw men at a distance coming to get other girls in the neighborhood. We ran to a nearby forest and hid for several hours.

When it got dark we ventured out of the woods, finally coming into a new neighborhood. We came to a house where there was a group of people who were helping to smuggle the girls out of the town to someplace safer. There were eight adults there, with a dozen or so girls of varying ages. We were all waiting for the van to come that would smuggle the girls out. We saw headlights coming, but the woman in charge said to hold the girls back and keep them out of sight. Sometimes the kidnappers drove by and she didn't want them to see the girls.

She went outside and started watering her flower garden. The lights drew near and she could see inside the vehicle that it was the people who had come to help get the girls to safety. She then told us to hurry and get the girls into the van before any of the neighbors saw them. All the adults were crying, hugging and kissing the girls goodbye. I hugged the two girls with me, looked them straight in the eyes and said that when this was all over I would come find them. I told them, "Be strong and take care of each other. I will come find you!"

## Interpretation

Although this dream seems like it is about human trafficking, it is also more personal to me. The story of the girls really helped me take a look at my earlier experiences and face for the first time the tremendous impact they had on me throughout my life. I was left by my mom and lived with my dad where others molested me. My innocence and trust were shattered. It made it very difficult for me to trust adults to protect me, especially men. It also closed off my willingness to feel any emotions on a deep level or let anyone get inside my protective wall so I wouldn't be hurt again. When my daughters were born, I was happy but unable to feel real joy and excitement. When other milestones were reached—graduation, our daughters' weddings, the birth of our grandchildren, the loss of a job—I reacted to these events and situations only on the surface, not with any depth of feeling. Through consciously forcing myself to stop and be present in the moment, I have become much better at really experiencing my life in all of its fullness, both good and hard times.

The role I played in the dream was also a great representation of the healing God was working in my life. Instead of being one of the victims, I was an adult helping the girls to escape the predators. I was confident and determined to find them and bring them back to their mom when it was safe. It produced in me the desire to help others who also had been wounded, either physically, emotionally, or both. This is something I hope to pursue when I retire. There are several women's shelters close-by to me and a group that works with those who have escaped from human trafficking situations.

## March 20, 2011—Stopping Perpetual Predators

In my dream, Ben had left to go home, but he snuck back into the house and came to my room where he raped me then left again. A few weeks later I found out I was pregnant. I was horrified, but I had to keep the baby. It was not the baby's fault. It was a little girl and I raised her by myself.

When she was a teenager, she told me Ben was so nice to her and took her to fun places. I warned her to stay away from him, that he was trouble, and his only interest in her was to have sex. She said I was wrong, that I didn't know what I was talking about, and stomped off to her room.

One afternoon a couple of months later she came to me crying and said I had been right. Since she had intercourse with Ben, he wouldn't have anything to do with her. I hugged her and told her it would be okay. Then she discovered she was pregnant. I said, "Great, he has fathered three generations: me, my daughter, and now her baby!" When he found out she was pregnant, he wanted her to come live with him. I told her she shouldn't go because she would just be one in a long line of other girls. He wouldn't take care of her while she was pregnant or take care of her baby. I begged and pleaded with her, but she moved in with him anyway.

The dream changed and it felt like I was watching a television show, detached from the action that was happening. In the show, my daughter had come back home with her baby because Ben had repeatedly slapped and punched her and she was afraid for the baby. She and I attended a school play, and Ben was in the audience at the back of the auditorium. At intermission I went over to him and asked what he was doing here. He said he came to take back what was his. I told him to stay away from my daughter or I would get a restraining order.

Then the television program changed and my daughter and I were at a fancy banquet for a local charity. Ben walked in and approached our table. I told him to leave, but he said not without the baby. My daughter told him he would never get the baby. He just laughed at us. I told him to leave or I would call the police. He said okay, she could keep the baby if we gave him $100,000 in cash right now. I told him we didn't have that kind of money, but we could try to get it tomorrow. He said, "Sorry, this is a one-time offer." He laughed again and said now he was sure he would get the baby because he could tell the court I had just agreed to pay money for the baby.

When he finished talking, my daughter stepped forward, with Nick and Scott on either side of her. She held her head up high, looked him straight in the eye and said he would never get the baby because the police were going to arrest him on multiple counts of rape of underage girls and impregnating them. He would spend the rest of his life in prison. The police came in then and led him away in handcuffs.

## Interpretation

Ben sneaking into the house and raping me was a constant fear that I lived with because of the lewd and suggestive comments he made to me. I wasn't confident that Mom would stand up to him and stop him.

In warning my daughter to stay away from Ben, I was trying to protect her the way my mom should have protected me. When I tried to tell Mom of my fears about him, she just treated me as if I was being foolish and silly, not taking me seriously.

Ben coming to the dinner to claim what was his showed how he felt he owned Mom. There was nothing she could do without asking him first. We were trapped in this lifestyle because we had nothing of our own; everything came from him.

The daughter stepping forward and facing Ben was, at least in my mind, a picture of me as an adult standing up to him and seeing he paid for what he had done. I was making sure he was stopped so he could never prey on anyone else. Although I was never able to say these words to him in real life, the fact that I was confronting him in my dream signaled I had conquered the fear of him and it brought a sense of peace to me that the cycle would stop here.

## February 22, 2012—Decision to Make Life Changes and Fight for Intimacy

I was at a college and picked up lunch from the cafeteria to take back to my dorm room to study. I ran into a friend who had been a missionary in France and asked him what he was doing here. He said he and his wife were in their last year as dorm parents for the high school academy associated with the college. He asked me why I was here, and I said Nick encouraged me to finish my degree, so we moved back here. Then we parted and I went to my room and put my lunch on the counter. The thought then occurred to me, "If Nick and I are here, why am I in a dorm and not married housing?" I left my room and went to the administration office to switch my living quarters.

A woman from the housing department showed me where the married housing was located and gave me a key. The key had numbers and letters on it (B3D)—letters for the building, numbers for the floor, and letters for the apartment.

I found the building, but couldn't make sense of the numbers and letters on the key. I stopped a student in the hallway, showed them my key, and asked if she knew where the apartment was located. She helped me find it and took me inside to show me around. There was a large living room with couches and chairs in red and gold brocade fabric and a big fireplace made out of rocks from the nearby river. Next to the living room was a large kitchen with new appliances, lots of cupboards, and an island for extra counter space. Around the corner from the kitchen was the master bedroom. It had a four-poster bed with lace curtains, a large armoire, and a window seat.

Connected to the bedroom was the master bathroom. It was all done in marble tile and had a big jetted tub and separate tile shower. There was also another bedroom and bathroom for guests down the hall. I thanked the student for her assistance and left.

I wandered around campus trying to think. I knew I had to make a choice whether to stay back at home with Nick and get on with my life there or for us to stay here and finish my degree. It would be a big disruption in our lives and Nick's job for us to stay here. However, I wondered if I could find a job back home without a degree.

I came upon a group of women swimming in a small pond. I joined them for a little while but none of them seemed to notice me so I continued on my way. Walking along a cement path, I saw a group of people who were sledding down a snowy hill and having a snowball fight at the bottom. They all looked at me funny, and I realized I was completely naked but not cold at all. They did not say anything to me, so I just walked past them and slid down the hill on my bottom.

The scene changed and there was a woman shriveled up like a ball on a couch. I was talking to Nick about her as if I were her therapist (she was really me). I told him she could come back, but it would take time and he had to do his part of nourishing her spirit, giving her encouragement, and building her confidence.

As I touched the woman she turned into a tiny worm in my hand. I brought her to him and told him he needed to talk to her and encourage her to grow. As he touched her and talked to her she did begin to grow and formed a head on one end. I told him he needed to teach her how to come back to become the woman she was meant to be. He put the worm in his hands and caressed it and spoke encouraging words to it, causing the worm to grow again. It kept growing until it became a full-grown woman. I encouraged the woman to try making love with Nick when they returned home. She was hesitant at first, but she was also excited by the new feelings that were stirred up in her. As I talked to them a few weeks later, they were both ecstatic about the level of intimacy and joy they were experiencing in their marriage.

## Interpretation

I was trying to bring closure to my past by wanting to finish my degree. I believed I needed to finish it in order to be complete as a person. Although it was not true that I had to finish, that was my perception of my life at the time. I was not looked on favorably in job interviews without a bachelor's degree even though I had two associate degrees and thirty years of experience.

I was also grieving the loss of having to quit the veterinarian technician program because I had broken my foot and had to have surgery. After the foot healed, I was not able to work in the clinic on my feet for ten hours a day without severe pain. I was not pursuing the career I wanted, and I felt stuck in a part-time job. I had been so focused on me and what I wanted that I had been neglecting Nick.

The married housing was a beautiful place. It was similar to the house we now live in which God gave us to enjoy and use for His glory. We have been blessed to have many friends and family members stay with us on their journeys to other places. It reminded me that Nick and I *choose* to share a wonderful life together.

The dream was not really about choosing between Nick and a career. It was about choosing to be happy with Nick and what we have or strive for a degree and a career that put us both under stress. I was trying to seek counsel from others to make a wise decision about pursuing my degree, but no one wanted to listen, like the women at the pond.

Being naked in the snow expressed my vulnerability in opening up to others and sharing with them my struggle of my sense of worth being tied to a degree and a better job. I believed other people judged me because of what I did as my job instead of who I was as a person. I wanted to make my decision based not on other people's expectations but on what was best for Nick and me and what I was physically able to do as a job. Of course, the biggest problem was trying to decide this myself instead of discussing it with Nick and hearing how he felt about both options. I forgot that being married is a partnership where both people have a say in what affects their lives together. I also was not asking God what He wanted for me. Once I had talked with Nick and prayed about the situation, I was able to decide to quit pursuing the degree and find a great job I love.

The end of the dream symbolized my newfound perspective of sex and intimacy as God intended it to be between a husband and wife. It was a journey that took time, patience and encouragement, but ultimately after many months I was able to participate and enjoy sex and intimacy with Nick in a much fuller way. I had to grasp hold of and cling to the fact that intimacy as God designed it was not bad or dirty. I had to let go of the shame and guilt I had associated with marital intimacy for such a long time.

By talking with Nick and my therapist, and reading what God says in the Bible about love, I learned to see it as something God gave me to enjoy with my husband in a way that truly makes us one. I couldn't have reached this point of freedom and wholeness without Nick's patience and encouragement to go at a pace that was comfortable for me. Although I know it frustrated Nick at times, for me it was a picture of sacrificial love that he would be content with the level of intimacy I was able to offer and not push me for more than I could realistically give.

## March 24, 2013—Conquering Fear and Helping Others

There was a family consisting of the parents, an older daughter, Sheila, who was sixteen, a son, Tom, who was thirteen, and a younger daughter, Donna, who was ten.

One day the mom gave the kids boxes and told them to start packing up everything in their rooms because they were going to switch bedrooms. The parents were trading rooms with Donna, and Sheila and Tom were switching rooms with each other.

As they were packing up, Donna's behavior began to change. She would have emotional outbursts, with screaming, yelling, and sobbing. Her parents did not know why she was acting this way or how to deal with her. Donna was throwing her toys, striking things with her hands and shouting that she did not want to move from her room to her parents' room. This behavior went on for a couple of days. When her mom confronted her and asked why she was so upset, Donna opened her closet and dresser drawers, pulling out her clothes and toys: "I don't want to go through all of these things and pack them," she said. So her mom helped her pack up her room, explaining that Donna did not have to get rid of any of her things, except for her radio. At the mention of her radio, Donna grabbed it and sat down on the floor, hugging it tightly while rocking back and forth mumbling, "No, no."

The week before the move, the mom hired an interior designer to help her with decorating ideas for everyone's new room. Donna became more hysterical and acted out as the time for the move approached. She kept screaming she did not want to move. One day the designer had enough of Donna's crying and asked Donna why she was upset about moving. The designer told Donna she would design a beautiful bedroom for Donna with princesses and fairies on the walls. Donna kept crying and said her parents were not letting her take her radio to her new room, but the radio was what helped her drown out the bad things. When the decorator asked what bad things, Donna said mommy is always crying and screaming and daddy makes grunting and growling noises. She was afraid if she moved into their room then someone would hurt her like they hurt mommy.

The designer told the parents what Donna had said. The mom replied that Donna was being silly; no one was getting hurt. Besides, Donna was always asleep by the time they went to bed and made love. The designer suggested they might talk to a counselor about Donna's fears. The parents went to a counselor and told him what had been happening. He said that what Donna was feeling was not uncommon, and he had seen it many times in working with children. Kids hear more than we think they do, but they have no context to interpret what they are hearing. To Donna's mind, the threat of harm to her mom and to her was very real.

## Interpretation

Donna's anguish mirrored how I felt when I heard Mom and Ben having sex. I thought she was being hurt and it terrified me. I had already lost one parent, and I was afraid of what would happen to me if I lost her also. When I finally confronted Mom about how I felt, she gave me the same response that the mom in the dream gave to the decorator, that I was just being silly. Only my mom did not talk to anyone else about it, she just told me never to mention it again. So I lived with the fear that I might wake up one morning without her there, at least until I was old enough to know what was really happening in Mom's room.

Donna's outbursts and acting out were pictures of me when I lived with my dad, wanting someone to see what was being done to me, because at four years of age I didn't have the words to express what happened. I also might have been afraid that I would get in trouble for telling or that they would say it was my fault. Hearing the noises from Mom's room may have triggered memories of those times when I was molested and it renewed my feelings of being helpless to stop what was happening.

The idea of switching rooms represented my anxiety that Ben's passes at me would lead to something more. I was very afraid he would trade Mom for me and I would have to trade my bed for hers.

The designer was a picture of me reaching out to protect and comfort Donna with my perspective now as an adult. It helped me see that I was getting better at dealing with the trauma in an appropriate and mature way. I wanted to help her understand that no one was being hurt. It was what I wished someone would have told me to take away the constant uncertainty for so many years.

Mom's response that I stop being silly and not speak about it again reinforced the message from her that my feelings were not important or valuable, and they were not to be expressed. I was still taking second place to Ben.

God was moving me to show compassion to other victims of abuse. I wanted to let them know they were not alone in their struggle to feel loved and accepted. Most of all, they needed to hear that they had worth and value and that the abuse was not their fault. They did not have to feel ashamed for what happened. They needed to know God could heal them of the emotional, and sometimes physical, scars of abuse. He began planting the seeds for this book even back then.

I want to share the following because both writers used words that are so elegant and beautiful in describing something so horrible and disturbing. I found this written on a bathroom stall in the ladies' room at a gas station.

The first three stanzas are part of the lyrics from the song "The Severed Garden" by The Doors. The last stanza was written by someone in a public bathroom stall. I felt like this was her cry for help. I prayed that God would provide the person who wrote this with some kind of assistance for her situation, someone she could talk to or who could rescue her. There are many, many more out there just like her. Please pray for them all.

## "The Severed Garden" by The Doors[1]

They are waiting to take us into the severed garden
You know how pale, wanton, thrillful
Comes death in the strange hour
Unannounced, unplanned for
Like the scary over-friendly guest you brought to bed

Death makes angels of us all and gives us wings
Where we had shoulders smooth as raven's claws

No more money, no more fancy dress
This other kingdom seems by far the best
Until its other jaw reveals incest…

It brings us to the place of pain
But amid the yearning for flowers
The only things that saves us is
Obedience to the King of the garden

[1]  THE SEVERED GARDEN (AKA ADAGIO)
Words and Music by THE DOORS
© 1970 (Renewed) DOORS MUSIC CO.
All Rights Reserved
Used By Permission of ALFRED MUSIC

# 7

# Depression—Part I

## October 3, 2004—Trying to Find Order in Chaos

I was taking people who were in wheelchairs from church to church, looking for the place where a special concert was to be performed. No one we asked could help us find our way. When we finally found the church, I asked several people for a copy of the program, but no one would give me one. A woman said she had a copy, but it turned out to be from a previous concert. Because the people in wheelchairs created too much of a distraction, the usher told me we had to leave.

The scene changed and I went to see a new movie. I parked way in the back on the side of the building because the parking lot was so full. It was rather dark along the side of the building and I had a long walk to the entrance. When

I entered the theater lobby, a little child was with me and the movie was about to start.

While watching the movie, I had the sensation that the lead actress was me, like watching yourself from far away. I worked as a nanny for a widower who had four children. I was asking how their day had been and dishing out pizza for dinner. Later when I was tucking the youngest children into bed, they still had their toys with them. I gently took the toys away and told them it was time to go to sleep. Each one of the little ones got a kiss as they snuggled under the covers. I left the room and went down the hall to check on the older children, who were all settled into bed. One of them wanted a drink, and I went into the widower's bathroom to get some water. The bathroom was very masculine in décor, done in chocolate brown with forest green towels. The shower curtain was a plain sheet of the same green. I liked the smell in the room. However, it was completely devoid of any feminine touches and I thought it could use a few, such as curtains on the window and pictures on the wall. I took the water to the child and then returned to the kitchen to clean up.

The next day I went out the front door to call the children in for lunch and saw them with a bad crowd of kids who were smoking and cussing. I told my children to come home and that they were not allowed to hang out with these older kids. I entered the house, noticing it was very crowded inside. There were three different living areas with couches, chairs and fireplaces. Around the corner was the widower's bedroom with a sitting area, but it was open to the other rooms, with no walls or doors.

I was thinking of how to change the rooms to be more centralized and what pieces of furniture could be given away. The focus of my plan was to create a dining area where everyone could eat together. Currently, it looked like a cafeteria with an assortment of tables and chairs scattered in one part of the house. I looked out the window and saw it was dark outside. In horror, I realized I had spent all day and into the night envisioning the changes to the living spaces. Meanwhile, everyone had gone through their day without me. I ate dinner and went to check on the children before I went to bed. They were already asleep.

The children wanted to adopt a dog, and we went to the shelter to look for one that was good with children. They didn't have any that would fit our lifestyle, so we started back home. As we approached the house, an evil-looking man was standing between us and the house. He said I had to choose whether to go help less fortunate people in the world or come back to the house and my "one true love." If I came back to the house, the poor would continue to suffer in their poverty, but if I left the house for the people, the widower would die. However, to get back to the house I would have to pass by the evil man.

The scene changed and the widower and I were getting married. We had a happy life raising the children. Later, when he was dying, I sent for all the children to come say goodbye. I told them nothing was more important than family and extended family. That was the end of the movie.

I was so moved by the movie. I had a very deep feeling of contentment and hope (something I was not able to feel when I was not asleep). I couldn't wait for the movie to come out on video so I could watch it again and again. As I tried to leave the theater, my eyes would not stay open and it was very hard to see. I stumbled around looking for the exit and ended up at the cast party with all the actors from the movie. I kept telling everyone how awesome the movie was and the little child was with me again. We walked around the set looking at the props and meeting the actors. I told them how much their role and the movie meant to me. I took the child around the corner and her favorite actor, the person who played the widower, was there. We started to back up out of the way, but he said it was okay and we came over to meet him. He talked to the child and gave her a bag of toys from the movie. She asked if he had a picture of him, but he didn't have one with him. The cast was going to take a group picture. I took the child up front with the other actors to get in the picture. I went to pick up my purse from a chair and while I was gone they took the picture. The little child waved so I could see her. We then collected some souvenirs from the movie set, thanked everyone for their graciousness to us, and got ready to leave.

Suddenly, my hand was shaking uncontrollably. I couldn't stop shaking or see my surroundings clearly. I tried to reach out and touch what I was seeing, but my eyes wouldn't focus. I ran into some cast members who were giving the child some brownies. The child was playing with the dogs from the movie. We finally managed to find the exit and get back to our car. I talked about the movie the entire way home, about how impressed I was by its message. As we drove away from the theater, I saw children from the movie tearing down a pool. I told them what a waste it was to tear it down, because we would have to spend next summer rebuilding it and finding water to fill it. It would be very hard work to do in the heat of summer.

## Interpretation

Going from place to place with the people in wheelchairs represented the struggle to find help in my depressed state. Some people offered the kind of help they thought I needed, but it was not the right type for me. Unfortunately, the church as a whole was not a source of help for me, even though some people in it supported me with understanding and encouragement.

As a nanny, I was trying to take care of my inner child by protecting the children from harm and nurturing them. The wall I had subconsciously erected in my emotions when I was a small child to keep out the confusion and trauma needed to come down. My therapist said I was a good mom to my children and I needed to help this "child" inside grow up to adulthood emotionally.

The part about spending so much time thinking about how to redo the house reminded me that sometimes I get so caught up in "my world" that I forget about others around me. Focusing on my depression caused me not to be present emotionally in moments with my family. Their lives kept going and I missed out. It also was a picture of trying to bring order out of the chaos that I felt in my mind and emotions.

The passage about having to choose between the widower and the world represented choices I was making or needed to make and how I felt about the decision-making process. I had to decide to move out of depression or stay where I was. I could change some things that triggered the episodes of depression or I could give up and spiral further down into a deeper depression. I had learned that choices have both good *and* bad outcomes. I was feeling good about making some hard choices that required me to fight back because I knew they were the right choices for me. I also learned that I have to take ownership of my bad choices such as giving into the pull of depression and curling up in a ball, missing time with my family and friends. God also showed me I can enjoy good things in my life.

The child meeting the cast members mirrored the little girl in me being able to find good people to believe in. She was shown kindness and felt included by being part of the group picture. I, however, was left out of the picture. I missed being included by others in my life, although sometimes it was a result of my own choices or my focus on my depression and missing the opportunities to join others.

Tearing down the pool pictured for me that sometimes we have to tear down things in our lives that are hindering us from making room for new and better things. However, both the tearing down of old things (habits, choice patterns, etc.) and the building of new things (focus on God, loving myself, living in Christ's freedom) takes hard work that can be messy and painful. I now know that no lasting change in our lives can occur without our choice to let God work in us to bring His peace and healing.

# December 17, 2004—Looking for God in the Church

I was driving a long distance and feeling very alone. I stopped and went to a church where a group of people were gathered in the foyer. They pretty much ignored me; no one welcomed me or spoke to me. The pastor was asking for someone who would paint the handicapped spaces in the parking lot. I asked him if I could do it, but someone else came along and did the painting.

I went back inside and hung up my coat on an outside hook of the coat rack. I entered the sanctuary and then came back out to the foyer to move my coat to an inner hook to allow people coming in late to have the outside hook. I went back to the sanctuary, but the usher said I was too late, the service had started, and I couldn't go in. I felt extremely depressed. I was hardly able to move or face anyone. I tried to go in at the beginning of each service but I could never get in before they closed the doors.

After the last service, a group of adults and children were singing in the foyer. I realized everyone in the group were either missionaries or worked for missions organizations. Still, no one talked to me. I went outside where tables and chairs were set up all over the lawn for a picnic. Nick was already sitting down, but there was no chair at the table next to him. I found a folding chair lying in the grass nearby. Since no one offered to help, I brought the chair to the table myself and sat down next to Nick.

Later during the picnic, I tried talking to a friend about what I was feeling, but she couldn't understand what I meant. I had a deep feeling of anger and of being alone. I felt scolded by people for being in the way and hopelessly unable to connect with another person. If this is how the church deals with broken, hurting people, then I'll pass. I didn't want to talk to God or have anything to do with Him.

## Interpretation

I was at the beginning of a long journey through depression. I looked to my church for love and help in dealing with the upheaval in my life. However, I was still pushing back at God as my source of help and felt that neither He nor the church wanted me.

Most people feel uncomfortable around those who suffer with depression. They are sympathetic for a little while but then make you feel as if they are thinking, "Get over it and be cheerful again." They aren't able to understand what it feels like not to have the energy to put the dishes in the dishwasher or take a shower or even eat a meal unless someone reminds you to do it.

I was trying to be helpful and considerate with the painting and the coat hooks, but I was not allowed to be useful. Because my therapist had me stop all activities I was involved in, except for going to work and to church, I was feeling adrift and unattached after being so busy with activities in the church before. I felt guilty for my family to have to carry my load at home. I wanted to help, but the depression robbed me of the energy to do even simple tasks. The reference to people in missions meant I hadn't lost my desire to serve others, but I was still struggling to function in a group setting.

The part about the chair at the picnic was about my feelings that there was not a place for me and others wouldn't help me fit in. It was also about my feelings of not being included by others, even though I had things to offer. I still had ideas and comments, even if I could not physically or emotionally carry them out, but other people felt too uncomfortable around me and didn't want to hear me.

## February 25, 2005—Feeling Lost in Depression

I was working in a government office, like an embassy, in some Asian country. I enjoyed my job and my coworkers. Suddenly one day, men dressed in black with faces covered and guns raised, stormed the embassy building and started shooting into the air. I grabbed three children of staff members who were in the next room and took them into a small closet. After the shooting stopped, we came out, and I found the other embassy personnel were still alive. We were all led away by the gunmen to a building by a wide, dirty river. The water was brownish in color, with sewage and garbage floating near the shore. The captors didn't like us being in their country, and they put our group on a platform that resembled a raft tied together with ropes. The bad men put all of us onto the raft and put it into the river, sending us off into the raging water. The river had a rapid current that tossed the raft up and down, and many of the people fell off and drowned.

The scene changed. I was still overseas but in a different part of the same country. The military patrolled all the streets with guns drawn. The soldiers said all foreigners had to get out of the country, but we couldn't get flights until the next day, so everyone had to find a room for the night. There were no hotels in the city, only rooms for rent in people's houses or hostels. Everyone was scrambling to find a house that had a room available. I found a house and was the first person to ask for a room. The owner gave me a room right away. As I was waiting for my room key, a lady came in and said she would like to stay in the Palm Tree room. The name of the room was vaguely familiar but I couldn't place where I heard it before. Suddenly, I remembered a missionary friend had told me that if I was ever in this town, I should stay in the Palm Tree room. She said it had the most gorgeous view looking out above everything in town, and the sunsets were unbelievably gorgeous. I asked the owner if I could stay in the Palm Tree room also. He said yes and had a bellboy take me upstairs. The bellboy opened the door to a room and stepped aside for me to enter. When I came into the room, it was dirty and had no furniture, only a mat on the floor for sleeping. I went out into the hall to tell him he had taken me to the wrong room, but he had vanished. I started walking down the hall to find the room for myself. The stairways were all like a maze. You could see other staircases, but you couldn't get to them. I kept trying every stairway I could reach. Some of them would come to an abrupt end at a wall. Finally, I heard the voice of the woman who asked for the Palm Tree room. I had to climb over some big pieces of furniture in the hallway to get to the room. When I finally reached the room, I told the woman that the bellboy had made a mistake and took me to the wrong room. She said others had already come in the room and there was no space left for me so I would have to leave. As I turned toward the door, the bellboy reappeared to take me to another room.

Before I left the Palm Tree room, I looked around to see the elegant gold wallpaper hand painted with green palm trees, white silk curtains billowing in the breeze coming through the window, and an ornate bed carved of light wood with a white lace canopy over the bed. Then I saw the most breathtaking sunset I have ever seen. The sky was awash in colors ranging from mauve, to cotton candy pink, to sunflower yellow, and finally a blaze of orange along the horizon. I sadly went back down to the lobby, but now all the rooms in the house were occupied.

I left the house and got on a train going to another part of the city. I noticed a man on the train who appeared to be an American from his clothes and accent. I asked him where he was from, and he replied that he used to live in Atlanta but now lived here in this city and worked for an American company. I told him about the soldiers and asked him where I could find a room. He didn't know of any place in the immediate area, but he warned me to stay away from a certain section of town. He said the homes looked like hostels, but they were really brothels, and it would be very dangerous for me to go near there. As we got off the train, I asked him what this place looked like so I could stay away from it, but I couldn't hear his response as he turned and left. I was scared of being alone in this strange place with nowhere to sleep. Then I realized I didn't have any money with me, just my plane ticket.

## Interpretation

The robbers represented the depression trying to steal my happiness. I was enjoying being with other people and feeling productive, but the good feelings were ripped away from me when I least expected it. Grabbing the kids and protecting them was me trying to protect myself when I felt vulnerable around other people. If I felt they were unaccepting of my struggle with depression, I would retreat back to my corner of emotional isolation.

Even though some of the people on the raft fell off and drowned, I was not one of them. So far I had managed to escape drowning in my depression. It gave me hope that I could get better eventually.

The rooms in other people's houses represented being at the mercy and compassion of others from outside to help me when I could not function to think clearly or do simple tasks for myself. It was truly humbling to see their love in action for me and my family through their help with errands and their prayers.

The missionary, the Palm Tree room, and the sunset were symbols of the Holy Spirit pointing me back to God as my true place of refuge and help. It was a tiny glimpse of God's goodness, safety, and light. However, I was not yet at a place where I could let God have control of my life.

Following every stairway in the jumbled layout of the house and climbing over the big pieces of furniture to get to the Palm Tree room represented my perseverance in looking for a way up and out of depression. Even when I faced failure and dead ends, tackling the obstacles that were in my way to reach the light of the sunset was a huge step forward.

The statement that there was no room for me and not being allowed to stay in the Palm Tree room represented my attitude when I had been around some people. They seemed uncomfortable and not sure what to say or how to interact with me. They were not always patient with me when I was unable to stop being overwhelmed by simple things or when I couldn't participate in a group activity because of the depression. However, in my self-centered, self-preservation existence then, I must confess I was not very patient or understanding with them. It was easy to have a pity party and see only my problems. But I have learned through this journey that everyone has a story that shapes who he or she is, and I need to extend the same grace and love to others that was shown to me or that I wished to receive from them.

Not having any money with me was an image of the insecurity in being equipped to handle the depression by myself. I did not possess the resources needed to lessen the grip of depression within myself. This realization was a first step toward admitting that I had to receive the help others offered. It also was the beginning of my path back to God. I needed to surrender control of my situation and trust God to be the provider of all the things I needed (through His Word, the Holy Spirit, professional therapists, friends, and family) to become the healthy person physically, spiritually, and emotionally that He created me to be.

## May 28, 2005—Facing the Reality of Depression

I was in the front yard of my house talking to one of the neighbors and she was upset because she thought I was going to make big changes to the outside of the house. I told her I was not changing anything on the house because I was only renting, I didn't own the house. As I was taking luggage out of the car, I noticed some construction workers next door. I was all alone in the driveway, and I wondered where the neighbor had gone. The workers were loading their equipment in their truck because the sky had grown dark with ominous gray clouds and the weather was getting bad. The constructions workers came over to my car and tried to kidnap me in their truck, but I ran away down the street, crying out for help.

The fire chief's car pulled up and a Scottish man told me my family had been in an accident. They were okay but they were taken to the hospital. I kept saying, "I want to see my family." He took me back to my car, a Volvo wagon, and I was glad to see the workers had left. The weather was turning very dangerous, with lightning and thunder and strong winds blowing debris down the middle of the street. We needed to get to somewhere safe. Inside the car were a lot of people of all different ages hiding underneath the luggage and blankets. I couldn't find our two dogs and had to leave without them. In the car with me were two babies, two small girls, four teenage/college girls, four teenage/

college boys, a husband and wife, and two single women. I met the Scottish man again and he had found our two dogs, two more lab puppies, and a baby. I put them all in the car and kept driving.

We stopped at a house, but my vision seemed cloudy, and I could not see the features of the house clearly. As I got out of the car, I could see that we were back at the same house we left earlier. The neighbors had bought the house for us. I was so excited. It had a little pool area and a stream with a strong current that gurgled as it flowed behind the house. Everyone in the neighborhood came and welcomed us. I was sitting around talking with them and kept saying, "God brought us back to where we started, but we had to go through the storms and trials to get here." As I was talking with the Scottish man, we looked up and saw a magnificent sunset in the distance, filling the sky with streaks of mesmerizing hues of purple, pink, and pale yellow. I thanked the Scottish man for his help and thanked God for this wonderful house.

I went into the house so we could see who would be in which rooms and get ready for bed. I was counting off who we had and how many would be in each room. I couldn't remember the names of everyone, so one of the teenagers helped me call everyone together. As I started up the stairs, I had a hard time walking and my hands felt numb. I tried to match people with rooms. I had four boys, but they didn't want bunk beds. I tried to decide which girls could room together. The boys didn't want to look at rooms and wandered off. I kept walking around and opening up doors to more and more rooms. There were big walk-in closets in each room and the master bedroom had a hot tub outside on the patio. The more I walked around, the more rooms and levels I found in the house. I kept getting confused who went in which room. I wanted the girls to pick their rooms with me, but they went on ahead to their rooms because I was too slow. As I worked my way downstairs, it kept getting darker. I was crying out for someone to come help me find the front door. Later Nick told me I woke him up talking out loud saying, "Hello, where is everyone?" over and over. When I finally got to the bottom of the stairs, there was a woman dressed in a business suit who said to me, "We need to go now." I told her I loved this house and didn't want to leave. She said that was the reaction everyone had. I looked back at the house as I rode away in the woman's car. Everyone and everything had vanished into thin air.

## Interpretation

Not making any major changes to the house showed I did not feel like I was making any significant progress in my depression. I could not make changes because I was not the owner of the depression; it was the owner of me.

The weather getting bad and the attempted kidnapping represented the dangers around me. It seemed like everything in my life was being taken away from me. I felt like I was in danger of slipping away from my life.

All of the people and things in the car was a picture of all the baggage of past losses I was carrying around with me: the losses of people who had died in my life, the death of our dog, the loss of our children being at home. I kept dragging those losses around with me instead of being able to let them go. Having to leave the dogs behind symbolized losing my sources of calm and joy. They showed me affection unconditionally even when I could not give it back to them.

It was interesting to me that the car was a Volvo. As a result of creative advertising, I connect the name "Volvo" with durability and safety. This was a place of refuge and safety for me. I was also fascinated by God's sense of knowing all of me in the reference to the Scottish man who helped me out. Although I did not know it at the time of the dream, I recently learned that my ancestors on my paternal grandmother's side were from a prominent family in Scotland. Maybe this is a symbol of how my family helped show me the way to safety and security.

The strong current in the stream visualized that some activities or patterns of coping might appear safe or desirable, but they were deceptive and dangerous, pulling me away from where I wanted to be. They might be comfortable, but they kept me trapped in depression.

God bringing us back to where we started referred to my fledgling belief that God is faithful and leads us and prepares us for what He has planned for us. I was "dipping my toes in the water" of having some trust in God.

The difficulty climbing the stairs and having no feeling in my hands represented my feelings of numbness and not being in control. I felt paralyzed with fear and so overwhelmed by all the tasks before me that it affected my ability to remember things or think clearly.

The boys and girls not wanting to look at the rooms with me was about my inability to communicate well to others what I wanted. My thoughts were not always coherent enough to talk to people, making it hard for people to have conversations with me.

The house opening up to more and more rooms described my journey of opening up to more and more things from the past and dealing with them in a concrete way, not avoiding them. But the depression made me confused and slow. I was crying out for help. Everything kept getting darker as I went deeper into the depression.

Losing the house at the end symbolized what I thought was perfect for me just fading away before my eyes. The job I had desperately wanted was taken away by a sudden medical condition. Things in my life were not what they seemed to be. I might have looked good on the outside, but I was a wreck on the inside. God was showing me that material things are fleeting and not satisfying. It was an idyllic picture of a perfect life, but it was not real. I had to deal with what life with depression really was instead of escaping into a fantasy.

## July 3, 2005—Facing the Past

I was fixing lunch for Nick, my friend, her toddler, and myself in the kitchen of a cabin. We needed to leave soon so we could get out of the woods and off the back roads before dark. I finished lunch and went outside to load my van. We were traveling in two vehicles, with Nick driving one and me driving the other with my friend. After driving for a few hours, we needed to stop and feed the toddler. We went through the drive-thru at a fast food restaurant and got dinner. Nick did not stop to eat and he was much farther ahead of us, almost home. My friend and I decided to stop for the night at a hotel rather than to continue driving. I called Nick and told him our plans.

We parked next to the entrance of a small hotel, like the old motor courts, and went to check in at the front desk. The desk clerk gave me the key to room 115, and we took our suitcases into the room. As I was closing the door, a man jumped out from behind the drapes and grabbed me. My friend and her baby were in the bathroom. I called to her for help, but my voice was barely a whisper when it came out. I jabbed my elbows into the sides of the attacker, and when he let go of me, I kicked him in the groin and he stumbled out of our room.

I ran to the front desk to tell the manager what happened. He apologized profusely and said he would give us our room for free. I went back to the room and my friend and her baby were okay. I wasn't able to sleep much that night because I kept reliving the attack in my mind. The next morning I packed my suitcase and went out to load up the van, but it was missing. I went to the front desk, where a different manager was on duty, and reported that my van had been stolen. He said I should have reported it missing last night. I told him I didn't notice it missing until this morning. It was there when I went to bed last night.

I was very upset because we were moving and I had our belongings in the van, including our couch. The manager said he would call the police, but there was nothing he could do about it. I went back to the room and my friend and her child were gone. I looked through the room and around the building and then went to the lobby to see if she was waiting for me there. The clerk said she must have taken the van and left without me. Every time I went to the front desk there was a different clerk or manager. I could never talk to the same person twice. I called Nick and told him what happened and that I would rent a car and drive home. I went to the lobby and looked in the phone book for rental car companies, but the pages listing rental cars had been ripped out. The clerk said he found some of my belongings, but he would not tell me where he found them. Next door to the hotel, people had tables set up for a huge garage sale. As I looked at the different tables, I found my clothes, towels, even my couch for sale.

One of the hotel staff let me borrow a pickup truck, and I left to find a rental car company. Two cars followed me and tried to run me off the road. I was so shaken up that I came back to the hotel. The manager said he had found a vehicle I could use. A man drove up in a jeep, and I told him it was too small to hold all of my things. Finally, the manager drove out an old Packard that was stored in his garage and he said I could use it. I thanked him and said I needed to drive it home, unload it, and then I would bring it back. He said he would have to drive it and bring it back himself. I called Nick to see if he could meet us halfway and we could load the couch and the rest of the items into our truck.

All through the dream I believed the hotel staff was being dishonest and shady. Something suspicious was going on, but I didn't care. I just wanted to go home. I sat down on a bench in front of the building where we agreed to meet Nick and waited for him to arrive.

## Interpretation

The cabin out in the woods represented the isolation I felt. I was trying to get away from it before the darkness came. All the things in the van symbolized my baggage from my past. God was trying to release me from it, but I was frantically trying to get it back and keep it with me. I was not yet ready to let go of all that happened in the past.

Nick driving one vehicle and me driving a different car was like my relationship with my dad. He drove ahead of me when he left and we were separated for a time. I came back to him for three years and then I had to leave him and never see him again.

When the man grabbed me in the room I thought, "Where is my friend?" I couldn't understand why she wasn't helping me. She was in another room protecting her child, but when I was a child, no one protected me. No sound coming out when I tried to scream symbolized my desire to be heard and helped when I was a child, but no one listened or considered my voice to be important.

When the manager said he was sorry about what happened and offered to give us the room for free but did not give us another room, I thought we were being placated so I would stop bothering him. The danger was still present and lurking in the dark.

Having the van taken in the night meant I had no way to get away from the bad situation at the hotel. It was a picture of my childhood experience; I could not get away from the abuse as a child or from my mom's relationship with Ben. I was trapped until other circumstances intervened (e.g., leaving my dad or moving away to college).

The manager saying I should have reported the missing car sooner made me think of people saying I should have told someone about the sexual abuse. I didn't have the capacity at the age of four to know what was happening, let alone put it into words to tell someone else. Besides, whom would I tell? Would they believe me?

The van was full of the belongings we were moving and suddenly it all disappeared. When I left my dad, I had to leave everything behind—my toys, my doll, and my clothes. I came back to my mom with only the clothes on my back. In the dream, my friend and her baby being missing reminded me of how I felt when I came back to live with my mom. Everything in my life when I lived with my dad had just disappeared and would never be found again.

The rental car pages being torn from the phone book, as well as my being run off the road when I tried to find a rental car place, represented my search for help that seemed to be thwarted at every turn. Until I began therapy and found a safe place to explore my past, I believed no one was listening to me as my life spiraled out of control. Of course, this wasn't true. Nick knew for over a year that I needed to see a therapist, but you cannot make someone seek help if that person isn't ready to accept help.

The garage sale next to the motel had all my personal things being sold to strangers. They represented letting go of all of the junk I had carried around with me from my past and being free of the weight and encumbrance they held on my life. However, I was angry with the people selling my property and frantically tried to find a vehicle so I could continue to keep the past with me. It was scary to get rid of what was familiar and comfortable. In my journey through depression, I had no place to store this baggage; it had to be thrown away. I had to learn how to release it in a positive way. I could not change what happened but I could give the things in the past and their power over me to God so they did not continue to dominate my behavior.

Telling the hotel manager that I would drop off the rental car reminded me of my dad dropping me at the airport and abandoning me there. He didn't come on the plane with me. I flew halfway across the country alone with my leg in a cast. I had no memory of the mom who was meeting me at the other end. I hadn't seen her since I was two years old. I must have been frightened being at the mercy of strangers. I didn't know what life would be like living with her.

Waiting for Nick to come meet me and take me home symbolized the hope of rescue and safety. Nick loved me and he would protect me, not abandon me.

## August 25, 2011—The Difficult Journey of Letting Go

I was in a parking lot outside of a school building and the air felt as if a bad storm was approaching. The sky was turning darker and the billowing steel-gray clouds were piling up on top of each other as they blew across the sky. There were other people in the parking lot watching the sky. In the distance we saw a tornado forming out of a huge black cloud, moving closer and closer, heading right at us. We all ran into the gym of the school and huddled together in the locker room.

We heard the tornado outside but it did not hit the school directly. We could hear howling winds and some of the debris hitting the building, but the roof stayed intact. When the noise and wind finally stopped, we went outside to see what it looked like. Nothing had been severely damaged, just some tree limbs strewn around the playground, broken windows, and bricks that had come off the building.

After making sure that no one was severely injured, people headed for their cars to go home. I gathered up my backpack and a couple of bags of yarn and I got on a bus that the city had sent to take people to their homes. As the bus started down the road away from the school, we could see more storm damage. There were traffic accidents where cars had been thrown around by the strong winds and landed on top of other cars and buildings. There were many vehicles abandoned along the road where people left them to go seek shelter.

The bus continued up the road and I told the driver that we were close enough to my house that I could walk the rest of the way home. He stopped the bus and I got off with my bags and started walking.

After a little while my walking got slower and slower, and I noticed I didn't have one of my bags anymore. I came around the corner of a brick building and saw a large, two-story house and thought, "This is not the way home." I turned around and started going a different direction. As I kept going, it seemed like I could hardly put one foot in front of the other until I was almost at a crawl. I was tired, sluggish, and having trouble breathing. Ahead of me on the right was a dirt road that had several trailers parked side by side down the road.

As I approached the trailers, I saw someone in front of me who looked familiar. The person turned around and it was my mom. I called out to her, trudging toward her. She took me into one of the trailers and told me to lie down for a little while. After I rested, she said I could stay in the trailer next door because the people who lived there had moved away. I noticed my backpack was missing and I asked her what happened to my blue bag. She said I didn't have any backpack with me when I got there. I was frantic because my wallet was in that bag and now I had no money or identification.

We walked outside and I could see the devastation from the tornado everywhere around us. Trees were stripped of their bark and many were completely uprooted. We went into the trailer next door. It was filthy and the only furniture in the room was a broken-down couch with torn, faded green fabric on the cushions. I didn't care what it looked like because I was so tired I just wanted somewhere to sleep.

When I got up the next morning, I started walking down the road to see the other trailers and the people who had survived the storm. As I walked along, the road began to descend into a valley. It became more like a rutted path winding back and forth, strewn with rocks and weeds. I realized I had been gone quite a long time and I should start heading back to the trailer. When I got back, Mom was gone. I asked the people in the other trailers if they had seen her, and they said she had gone down the road with a large group of older people. I started running that direction in a panic. I finally heard her voice coming from outside a small building where other people from the trailers were huddled together. I raced to her and hugged her tightly. I was crying and told her I was afraid she was gone and I would never see her again.

## Interpretation

I survived the storm, which was the molestation when I lived with my dad. There was not much visible damage of the abuse in my life, other than wetting the bed and being afraid to have a bowel movement, but there was a lot of emotional damage under the surface.

Walking slower, going the wrong way home, missing a bag was all a picture of me when I began to deal with depression. The depression slowed me down and was taking me in the wrong direction. I was tired and worn out from carrying all the emotional baggage with me throughout my life. But the missing bag represented that I had started to let go of some of my old baggage.

In the dream Mom tried to take care of me by telling me to lie down and rest. In real life, she tried her best to provide me with all I needed and a good life as a child. But there was a clear divide. Her trailer was neat and clean, but I could not stay there emotionally. She had no room for me. I would stay in the dirty trailer next door with broken furniture. It resembled me when I came back to my mom at age five, literally filthy and emotionally broken.

Missing the bag with my wallet and identification represented how I came to Mom without any of my toys or favorite things, nothing but the clothes on my back. I had no real identity, no idea of who I was, and no memory of this woman that was my mother. I had been uprooted from my life with my dad and everything with her was strange and unfamiliar.

I had descended into a valley with all that happened in my early childhood, but I had a chance to make it back up the hill to a better life with Mom. Physically, it was much better. I had food, clothes, a safe place to live, and someone who took care of me. But when the dream refers to Mom going on ahead, it was like Mom emotionally going with Ben and leaving me behind. I was looking for that safe place emotionally. I was so afraid of losing her because if I lost her, I would have to move to another place with relatives I didn't know that well. It heightened my insecurity because I didn't know if the new place would be safe or more like my life when I lived with my dad.

## January 15, 2013—Fighting against Depression

While working at a restaurant waiting tables, there were several customers who were surly and rude. They kept heckling me and causing a commotion. Two other employees in the back room refused to come out and help me. More and more customers were coming back to the kitchen, disrupting business, and then they began pushing and hitting me. The manager came in from the back room, and I asked him to help me get all of these people out of the kitchen. He just said not to worry, it would be all right. I told the manager I couldn't work in a place where I wasn't protected and walked out.

As I left the building and started home, the people inside the restaurant started yelling and chasing after me. I ran faster and faster, trying to get home before they caught up to me. I could hear my heavy, labored breathing. In reality, I was tossing and turning in bed and talking out loud so much in my sleep that Nick got up and went to the guest bedroom. The next thing I remember was Nick rushing into our bedroom and shaking me awake, telling me I had screamed so loud that he heard me from the other side of the house.

I went back to sleep and fell right back into the dream. I reached home, and Mom was on the couch with two kids and she just stared at me. One of the children was a little boy and he climbed up next to me on the other couch and told me he would protect me. Suddenly all of the people that were chasing me burst through the front door of our house and piled on top of me, hitting and punching me. When they finally left, I stumbled out of the house, followed by the little boy. As I turned around I saw him standing in the middle of the street looking at a puddle. He looked at me and said, "She's gone. They killed her." Then I woke up.

## Interpretation

I was going through a period of depression where I felt battered, beaten, and overwhelmed with life, experiencing uncertainty in my job and with our finances. Our adult children were making choices that concerned us, and I was trying to share my concerns without telling them what to do. I found talking to them without making them feel disrespected as adults very difficult.

Kicking in bed was the physical acting out of the mental battle within. I was trying to beat off the depression, but it kept attacking me. Just when I thought I could see a little progress, the depression would seem to come out of nowhere and the emotions would overwhelm me to the point where I felt immobilized and unable to go to work or even get out of bed.

Mom on the couch with the blank stare, disengaged from the two children, was a picture of how I lived with my two girls. So many times when they were growing up, I was with them physically, but I could not be present with them emotionally. I didn't have the emotional energy to engage fully in what they were doing or sit down and play a game with them or read to them. My depression caused fatigue, making me too tired to help them with projects or homework. For many years I felt I had failed them as a mom. I didn't always give them my full attention when they needed it. I struggled to divide my time between the two of them and give each one what she needed. So often I was keeping myself too busy with life in order to keep the depression at bay and that busyness took away my time from them. I have talked about this with both of my daughters and asked them to forgive me. They said they forgave me and they always knew that I loved them. Their forgiveness meant so much in helping me to forgive myself and let go of the guilt I felt about not being present for them.

Sometimes the exhaustion, numbness, isolation, and loneliness of the depression was so hard, I felt as if I'd dissolved into nothing but a dirty puddle. I thought who I was before the emotional breakdown had died, and this was how life would be from now on. Eventually, as I prayed and received support from family and friends, these episodes began to be less frequent and I could see a glimmer of hope. I knew I could never go back to the life I had before because it was not normal or emotionally healthy, but I could reclaim the good things of my former self and go forward to become the person God was shaping me to be.

# 8

# Depression—Part II

## June 23, 2004—Facing Depression

I was in a classroom laughing with my friends, giggling uncontrollably. In my hand was a glass of fresh lemonade. Mark, my therapist, was teaching the class and he asked me if that was the same glass of lemonade I had in first and second period. I said yes. He went on with the class, when I blurted out, "What happens if I still have the glass in seventh period?" Mark said, "I don't know. What do you think should happen?" Then one of the other students asked incredulously, "You have this guy four times a day?"

The dream changed and I was in a different classroom, talking with my friends. I told one of them that I had to go refill my lemonade before seventh period. I went to the bathroom to rinse out my glass, and there was a girl sitting on the floor, just staring blankly off into space. I asked her if she was okay. She just kept staring without looking at me or answering. I asked her what was wrong. Another girl who was in the bathroom said, "Depression." Then the girl on the floor shook herself, said she was okay, gathered her belongings, and left the bathroom without saying anything else.

I was back in the classroom laughing with one of my friends when Mark asked if I would like to share what was so funny. I said no, gathered up my books, got up and left. On the way out of the building, I saw Sandy, a girl who was on the soccer team. She looked sad and I asked her what was wrong. She said her parents were out of town and she didn't have a place to stay for the night. Another girl, Lily, invited her to stay at her house, but Lily needed to check with her parents first. I told Sandy that if it didn't work out to go to Lily's, she was welcome to stay at my house.

## Interpretation

Mark, my therapist, was a safe person to joke with and let down my guard a little. He helped me learn to experience emotions again by having me identify emotions I had every day. In sessions, I could express the loneliness or fatigue or lack of hope I felt because of the depression. He gave me ideas of things that would help, like journaling and giving myself permission to do fewer activities when I was fatigued.

The references to carrying lemonade and having Mark as my teacher in four classes appeared because I always had a travel mug of coffee with me at our sessions. At the beginning of my therapy, I needed to see Mark once a week to be able to function at work and in daily life. In the dream, Mark and I were in a classroom setting because he was showing me how to be myself again and that it was possible to have fun again with my friends and family.

The part with the girl who didn't have a place to stay was an example of how I was beginning to feel compassion for someone else and reaching out to help others instead of being wrapped up in my own depression.

The girl in the bathroom illustrated me facing the fact that my mental health and lifestyle were out of control and declaring to myself the truth that I was suffering from severe depression. I could finally see how lost and empty I felt being disengaged from everyday life, and I was now willing to face it head on.

The reference not to tell Mark what was so funny actually represented the opposite. Although I was feeling at ease with Mark, I was not ready to tell him all of what was bothering me. I knew it would be hard to relive the situations I had been through, and I was not yet willing to experience the pain and sorrow that was emotionally connected to my past. I had kept them secret for so long that I was afraid to say them out loud to someone else.

## October 6, 2005—Wanting Out of Depression

I was driving my car down a country road when I saw an oncoming car in my lane. I swerved to avoid the car, went off the shoulder and down the embankment. I couldn't remember what happened afterward, but I woke up in the hospital and miraculously only had a sprained wrist and some bruises. A familiar-looking woman came to take me home, but something seemed not quite right. When I entered the house, the furniture and other items in the house either were not in their regular place or they were missing altogether. When I asked where my rocking chair was or who moved the living room furniture and the picture over the couch, the woman said I never had a rocking chair in this room and I just didn't remember how the furniture was arranged. She told me I must be mixed up from the accident. As the days went by, everything in my life seemed different, just slightly off, but my friends said I still was suffering memory issues from the accident.

One day I opened the bottom drawer in my desk and there was a yellow pad of paper with notes I had written in my therapy session about God and myself. I knew these notes were real, not part of what seemed mixed up in my mind. From that point on, each day I remembered tiny pieces of who I really was. A few weeks later I was walking down the street in town and a young man approached me, asking if I wanted to go home. I said yes, I definitely did. Somehow I knew this life I was living couldn't be my real life. Suddenly I saw headlights approaching and I swerved just in time to avoid the accident.

## Interpretation

The dream was about my life with depression. I was realizing that the life I was living was not my true self. I had to stop believing the lies I felt when I was depressed, such as not being good enough or not having the energy to do anything. There was a spark of hope that I could return to normal or real life.

Being depressed resembled my real life but was not actually the same. The people were the same, things looked the same, but I could tell something was just not right. Depression made things in my mind slightly off-center. Enough things were similar to my real life, but it confused me and made me doubt myself. People would patronize me as if I were a little forgetful or mixed up when I couldn't remember details about an event or what someone had told me the day before. However, deep down I knew this was not who I truly was. I was living just a shadow of my life.

At the end of the dream, my wanting to go home signified making the decision to deal with my depression head on. Coming back to reality in the car and avoiding the accident wasn't about escaping the depression. I was learning to avoid the things that made the depression worse. I began to recognize the symptoms when I felt overwhelmed, and I was able to make better choices about boundaries on my time and energy and discern what I was able to handle emotionally.

## March 4, 2011—Looking for Help

We were at our daughter's wedding. The bridal party was rushing around getting dressed. I was helping the little flower girl get dressed. All of a sudden I was unable to do simple things like pull up my pantyhose or get my dress on by myself. My hands could not grasp the buttons or the zipper. My speech was slurred and I was acting like someone having a stroke.

I called Nick to help me get dressed, but he could not come in where the women were getting dressed. I asked one of the girls in the room to help me, but everyone just looked at me like they were disgusted and walked away. I sat in the room while the wedding went on. I missed my daughter's wedding! I asked for someone to take me to the food table at the reception and help me get something to eat. A woman took me to the table, and I managed to get a couple of pieces of fruit on my plate, but when I turned around to get some of the cake, the woman helping me was gone. I took my plate with the fruit and shuffled off. I found Nick and told him how the woman just left me at the table. He said to stop complaining; at least I got something to eat, and he pointed at my plate.

After the reception, I went back to the dressing room to get my things before we left. Everyone seemed mad at me because I was so needy. They seemed uncomfortable around me because I walked funny and talked incoherently.

## Interpretation

Depression made me feel overwhelmed by everything around me. I could not take in all the information that came at me daily from work and home and process it. I felt paralyzed just thinking about the routine things that needed to be done each day, such as what to make for dinner or how to do a load of laundry. My mind and body seemed to shut down and refused to function correctly. The experience was like being a normal person trapped inside a helpless body.

In my journal after this dream I wrote, "God please help me to escape the 'weird body' feeling of my depression where my brain and body don't communicate with each other. I feel purposeless and lack any direction. Help me to set goals, even little ones, and get into a routine that helps me feel productive. Give me a vision for what is next."

The episodes at the wedding and reception depicted my dependence on others to help with even small tasks I did not have the energy or mental capacity to do myself. Sometimes my mind seemed foggy and I couldn't remember how to cook eggs or load the dishwasher. I would sit and cry because I felt so stupid and helpless. I knew people were tired of me being like this, always needing assistance to do simple chores or remember where to find my shoes. I believed, although it was not really true, that people were disgusted by my neediness. They just wanted me to hurry up and get back to normal so they could get on with their lives. Even my family, at times, were tired of carrying the weight of extra work around the house because I could not manage more than one task a day, such as folding a load of laundry and putting it away or wiping down the bathroom.

At work I had to concentrate very hard on remembering the information I was given and the tasks I needed to accomplish. By the time I got home, I was emotionally and physically drained. Sometimes I didn't even eat dinner. I just came in and went to bed. The irony of this pattern was that when I finally told my boss about my breakdown about six months later (because I was afraid I might lose my job or have to take a leave of absence), he said he never noticed anything was wrong, that the work I did seemed the same as my usual performance. So I guess I must have pooled all my energy to keep it together at work, but when I got home I crashed, with nothing left to give.

## March 12, 2011—Letting Change Happen

I was going to meet my friend Andrew at the train station and take the train with him out of downtown Atlanta. He missed the train, so I got off at the next stop from downtown. As I disembarked from the train, I saw Andrew go over across the tracks. I called to him and he turned and waved at me. I tried to walk across the tracks to meet him before the next train came. There was a wide chasm between the two tracks and I had to walk on a narrow steel beam to reach the other side. Some construction workers were working on the beam and I could not pass by them. I told them I desperately needed to get to the other side of the tracks. They were able to maneuver just enough for me to get by them. As I was getting close to the end of the beam, the next train came that was headed out from the city and Andrew boarded it. I made it across the track after the train departed and sat down to wait for the next outbound train. I looked at each train stop for Andrew, but I didn't find him.

Time passed and I often thought of Andrew, wondering where he had gone. One day I got off the train at a different stop from my usual one to go to a craft show set up near the train station. I walked around looking at the different craft displays, finding a large booth that had beautiful handmade wood furniture. As I was admiring a desk, I looked up and there stood Andrew in front of me. I almost didn't recognize him. His hair had grown long and he had a short, bushy gray beard. I hugged him and asked him what he was doing here. He said he had enough of the hustle and bustle of the city and decided to stay here and make furniture. He excused himself to wait on a customer. I browsed some more and then had to leave and catch my train home. I occasionally got off to see Andrew at his booth but he became elusive, like he was avoiding me. When I finally found him one day, he told me he had been avoiding me because he felt guilty for not waiting for me at the train station and then never contacting me later to tell me where he was living. I told him it was okay and that I was glad I had found him again because he was still my friend.

The scene changed and Andrew was now an old man. His handmade furniture had made him famous and he had been sought after by many people from all over the country to make furniture for them. When I found him he was in a little room in a shabby old brick building that was crumbling in spots. The hallway to his room had many doors and they all looked alike. Some of the room numbers were missing and the walls were dingy with years of stains from cigarette smoke. It smelled musty and moldy. The hallway was very dim because most of the lights no longer had bulbs that worked.

As I entered his room, he told me to shut the door quickly before someone saw him. Over the years he had developed an extreme sensitivity to light, which caused excruciating headaches. He could no longer make furniture because of the headaches.

Suddenly someone burst through the door shouting, "Here he is!" I told the person to leave him alone and I shut the door. Andrew said now he would have to find a new place to live because they would know where he was and continue to hound him. That night I helped him down the hallway, down two flights of stairs and entered a room that was much larger than the one he had before. I got him settled into bed. He was very frail and seemed like he would crumble into pieces. More people were now outside the building, and I went out and told them he was very weak and they needed to leave him alone.

## Interpretation

Andrew missing the train and the large chasm between the two tracks represented my feelings of missing connections with my friends. There was a large void in my life between my friends and me. Some of them were not as close and friendly as they had once been. It was not that they didn't care about me, but they felt awkward and uncomfortable because I took so long getting better. They got tired of me not being able to participate fully in events. I was sure they thought I should hurry up and get over this depression and get back into the regular routine of life.

The narrow beam, the long time I took to cross it, and encountering construction workers referred to the long journey back from depression, which was filled with obstacles and setbacks that I had to learn to maneuver around. It was very scary and precarious to cross back to a normal life.

Andrew disappearing was about his getting off the roller coaster of the daily train ride and fast-paced job and doing something else he loved to do. That was how I was feeling. I was tired of the long commute each day and I was not feeling productive at work. I wanted to do something that I loved to do, something that energized me.

Andrew as an old man was my depression. The hallway with many doors symbolized the many choices in front of me. Missing room numbers signified the uncertainty and the unknown of what was behind each door. Dealing with depression was a choice and still is today. I could give in to depression and let it control my life or I could acknowledge it and try to fight it. In finding Andrew the first time, I had decided to confront the depression, but I didn't get rid of it. Like stopping to see Andrew from time to time, I continued to come back to the depression over and over.

Andrew's sensitivity to light shows how depression keeps you in the dark, in the shadows of your life. It is very painful at first when the light does come into your darkness, but as the source of the depression begins to heal, you can adjust to the light.

Getting Andrew settled into another room was like putting depression in its place. His frailty refers to breaking the ties binding me to depression. It also represents how fragile and vulnerable I felt while I was facing changing attitudes in myself and letting go of bad habits and patterns that kept me stuck in depression.

## January 12, 2012—Growing Outside of Myself

The dream started with a young girl in a chemistry classroom. The teacher talked constantly and the girl was struggling to write down every word she said. The teacher was very hard on her students and usually only two-thirds passed her class.

One day the teacher was berating the girl for not keeping up in class and saying the girl was not trying hard enough. The girl had had enough of the pressure and told the teacher that because of spending so much time on this class, she didn't have enough time for her homework in other classes. She continued, "You keep pushing me about going to college. If I don't pass my high school classes with good grades, there won't be any college. Don't you get that?" This encounter really changed the heart of the teacher to see that she had put unrealistic expectations on her students. After that, the teacher did not push her students beyond reasonable levels of work.

When the teacher got married later that year, the girl attended the wedding and told the teacher that she had just received a $25,000 scholarship for college. The teacher hugged her and said she was so proud of how the student's attitude and hard work had paid off. There was an older woman who worked in the office at the high school who was also at the wedding. She overheard the girl's announcement of her scholarship. The older woman told the girl she was so happy for her and was also very proud of her.

Then the older woman left and walked home very slowly. She traveled through many diverse areas: a group of prostitutes on a corner, a Swedish community, a German community, and a Chinese community. As she walked along, a little boy joined her. He showed her the few coins he had to buy his supper. Soon the boy saw another little boy sitting on the sidewalk in tattered clothes and he gave the other boy one of his coins. Farther down the road they saw a blind man sitting on the corner, playing a clarinet. The little boy put another of his coins into the man's donation box. Then they came upon a disheveled woman with a little baby, and the little boy gave her two coins. When they got to the market, the boy picked out what he wanted for supper, just a little bun with a single piece of meat in the middle. When he went to get the coins out of his pocket, he realized he didn't have any coins left. The older woman was so moved by the boy's generosity to the others they met along the way that she said she would pay for the boy's meal herself. But when the shopkeeper heard the story, he waved them both on and told them not to worry about paying.

The boy went home and the woman continued on her way. As she got near to her house, a younger woman stepped up and tried to take the older woman's soup away from her, but the older woman struggled to hold onto her package. Suddenly a man came up to them, startling the younger woman, and she let go of the older woman and ran away. He checked to see if the older woman was hurt, and she thanked him over and over. He just smiled at her and walked on down the street.

## Interpretation

The first part of the dream reflected the financial pressure I was feeling since I was only working part-time. I was afraid that working full-time would be too much for me emotionally and would bring back the depression. I was trying to find a balance between finances and emotional health.

The little boy traveling through all the different neighborhoods, giving to those in need, even at his own expense, was a picture of me working at conquering my depression by looking at the needs of others around me and helping them instead of being caught up in my own little world. I was walking along in my journey, seeing others who were also broken and needed help. The boy gave away all he had to help others and was rewarded by the shopkeeper (God) with what he needed.

The older woman represented me walking with the little child in me and seeing the child grow into someone I wanted to become. I wanted to help others who were struggling, hurting, and feeling alone.

The attack by the younger woman was a picture of the depression attacking me when I was maturing in my recovery. It was trying to steal away the good things God had given me. But God, as the strange man, stepped in to stop the attack. In my journey I still faced dangers, but I knew God would protect me, save me, and provide everything I needed.

# September 6, 2012—Trying to Break the Grip of Depression

My family lived in a small house, and one day a woman knocked on our door and said she had always admired this house and wondered if she could see the inside. As I began to show her through the house, the house became larger than it had been before. I took her upstairs and told her there was an unfinished attic, but when I opened the door, the attic had beautiful rooms at each end of the space with old fashioned decorative crown molding around the ceiling. The sides of the open space were piled up with books and toys spilling off of bookcases. As we walked toward the other end of the attic, it was set up like an apartment with a small kitchen, table and chairs, bed and sofa. Through the door was a spiral staircase that led down to the backyard. As we descended the staircase, I could see the very large backyard. It had a pool, tennis courts, and a fire pit area, as well as a large barbeque and eating area. There was a separate building that had showers and restrooms for men and women, and a big hot tub sat outside next to the building. All of these amenities had not been there before. The yard had been a tiny patch of grass with a clothesline and small wooden shed.

We came back into the house and entered a family room with a table that could seat twelve people. She said she wanted to buy the house and would come back tomorrow to write up and sign a contract. I told her that she could rent out the space upstairs with the separate outside entrance to help pay some of the mortgage payment. After she left, my husband and I sat down and thought, "Wow, we weren't even thinking of selling the house." I never knew all those other areas existed here. I had no idea how much we should ask for the house. The next day the woman came back and we all signed the contract. She gave us a very good price for the house. We moved out and she moved in with her husband and five children. About three days after we moved to our new house three blocks away, I saw a glow in the sky. I said, "Oh my goodness. The house is on fire!" We drove back to our old house to see how much damage there was. The house now looked like an old Victorian house with rounded turrets on the corners. I went inside and the only part of the house that had burned was the bedrooms. There were no survivors of the fire. The rest of the house was completely intact. I went upstairs to the old fashioned room at one end of the attic and saw a painting on the wall of a man from a long ago era, who was the original owner of the house. Suddenly I heard a voice say, "You didn't think I would let anyone else but you live here, did you?" I screamed and started running toward the stairs. The walls and floor started breaking up around me and I saw flames coming from below me. I tried yelling, "Fire!" and screaming, "No!" but no sound would come out of my mouth. I woke up and realized I had said, "No!" out loud. Every time I closed my eyes, I went back into the dream with the fire. I got up out of bed and went to sit in the living room until I was sure I was fully awake. After an hour or so, I went back to bed.

I started dreaming again, only this time I was with a group of people and we were leaving in several vans from the same Victorian house as before. As we were loading up the vans, all the lights in the house went out. There was a sense of urgency and panic as we hurried to leave. We finally got everything packed and drove away. As we drove down the highway, the lights around us went out as we passed them, almost like they were following us. We pulled over and had the rest of our vans go ahead of us. All the cars and trucks in front of us were crashing into each other because they couldn't see where they were going in the dark. When we finally caught up to our other vans, we stopped and looked behind us. All of the lights in the town were out. It was completely dark except for the Victorian house, which was outlined in lights with a glow shining out of every window.

We finally arrived at the airport and tried to check in all of our bags. We had baby chicks, bunnies, goats, a llama, a pig, turtles, and a cow. The chicks and bunnies were not in a cage or box, and we were trying to round them up and give them to the agent. He said we had to have a certain certificate for the goats, pig, and cow to travel. We could obtain the certificate back at the main terminal. We would miss our flight if we had to go back there, but he wouldn't let us leave without the certificate, so we headed back to the main terminal. On our way back there was a steep hill we had to descend. Some of the group tried to slide down it, but it was not slippery and they tumbled down. We got our certificate at the main terminal and hurried back to our gate to gather the luggage together. There was a pile of small items such as shampoo, toothpaste, and extra batteries that were not packed, and I was handing them to different people in the group to pack in their bags. As we started to board the plane, I realized I didn't have my ticket. I went toward the door of the plane and they were closing it. I screamed for them to wait. I saw a man behind me pick up a ticket off of the ground and I could see my name on it. I told the flight attendant that I had dropped my ticket and the man behind me had picked it up. She said she would get it from him and that I needed to take my seat. I sat down next to my family and the plane started to taxi out onto the runway. It was very crowded on the plane with only a little room for the flight attendant in the aisle. As we reached the runway, all the lights on the runway and in the airport terminal went out. My family looked at each other and said, "Oh no, here we go again." The pilot said he was going to attempt to take off anyway and for us to be sure we were safely secured in our seats. He started down the runway with no instrument lights on in the cockpit. Just as the engines accelerated to take off, I woke up.

## Interpretation

The small house represented my life. Depression limited my activities and my social interactions. I didn't have the energy to do anything but go to work, come home, eat dinner, and go to bed.

The expansiveness of the house that I hadn't been aware of portrayed all the possibilities and opportunities that were waiting for me outside of depression. I couldn't even imagine a full, exciting life.

Selling the house and then having it drag me back in was a picture of how I tried to get out of the depression but it had too much of a grip on me. It was destroying everything around me in order to keep me captive. I tried to be with other people at picnics or at church, but when I did, it felt like the darkness was closing in and it gave me a sense of panic. In a large group of people, I was overwhelmed when I thought of talking to so many people and thinking of enough things to say. It took too much of my energy, which was already in short supply.

The crashes by the vehicles as we drove to the airport were the roadblocks to my escape from depression. I was able to get around them eventually as I continued therapy and started changing my lifestyle to cut out a lot of the busyness with unimportant things. Sometimes, however, everything seemed so dark, except for the house (the depression), which was an illusion of light and reality that drew me in until I was trapped.

The scene at the airport with all the animals and the obstacles to getting on the plane dealt with my sense of loss and grief. I loved animals and I was so excited to get to work with them at the veterinary clinic. But when I could no longer do my job because of my broken foot, I went down into depression again. It was like the steep slope at the airport. It was not an easy slide, but a bumpy tumble. The chaos at the airport showed all the confusion in my life— the feeling of so many loose ends and attempting to delegate some of my responsibilities to others instead of crippling myself by trying to do it all.

The lost ticket symbolized my perception of losing the ability to move forward out of depression. The man who found my ticket was God, who had the only way for me to get on the plane and away from the depression: through prayer, asking God to help me break free of the depression, and through my therapy sessions. I learned to recognize the signs that lead to depressive episodes such as being excessively tired and withdrawing from people. I began to make better choices about my lifestyle, making sure I was taking care of myself by resting when I needed to and keeping close to God in my daily Bible reading. I also asked a couple of close friends I could trust if they would keep me accountable for my choices.

I was able to get on the plane and start to leave depression behind me with help from my family and friends. I realized depression was still chasing me and there would always be a possibility of recurrence in my life, hopefully not as serious as this episode. But I chose to leave it behind and go forward, even when I couldn't see where I was going. Now I truly believed I could trust God with whatever was in my future. He had protected and rescued me in the past and He would be faithful to do so in the future.

# 9

# Dealing with Change and Loss

## March 27, 2005—Struggling to Let Go of the Past

I was in a dorm room sitting in front of a computer but not really working on anything. My roommate brought a dog from a shelter and said this was the dog I agreed to take care of. It was a beagle that was very well behaved but in need of lots of love and attention.

I met some other people from our hall in the dorm. My first reaction was feeling out of place because they were all so much younger. I had been there a couple of weeks but had not yet been to class. I couldn't remember when or where the classes were held. I had one on Tuesdays at 11:00, but I couldn't remember the name of the class or where it met.

One day I met a nice guy who was fun to be around and he seemed to understand my confusion with my classes. He helped me get a copy of my schedule. After that we went to pay for the classes just as the financial office was closing. It was the last day to pay tuition or I would have to drop out and start again next semester. I talked to the lady at the window and she agreed to let me pay before they closed. From there we went to the bookstore to get my books, but it was also closing. I talked the cashier into letting me get my books. It was time for dinner so we went to the cafeteria. I had never been there before and I couldn't figure out how to swipe my card to pay for the food. The guy showed me how and we went through the line for dinner, talking about where we were from and what majors we were pursuing.

I went to my Tuesday class and really liked it. The professor said he was glad that I finally made it to the class. I had another class on Wednesday where they were going on a wilderness hike. I arrived at the starting point for the hike and had sandals on, but everyone else was wearing hiking boots. They told me I didn't have the right shoes and I would have to get boots to go on the hike. I went to the bookstore and bought boots, then rejoined the class. Not long after we started, the trail began climbing up a steep hillside. It was raining heavily and everything was muddy. It was very hard to get my footing on the wet, slippery trail.

The scene changed again and this time I was on a cruise ship. A group of people, including me, were going together on a shore excursion. I didn't know any of the people in the group. We went on a boat to a remote area and hiked into a particular village where they had an outdoor market that sold many different kinds of handmade crafts, such as beaded necklaces, bracelets with shells, straw hats, and baskets. Although I didn't remember ever being there before, I must have been because the villagers called me by name. However, as we left the village, I was explaining to the group that the villagers had no other source of income. They were separated from the mainland and had to use whatever resources they could find to make the crafts they sold to the tourists. They used the money they made during the tourist season to live on the rest of the year.

Back on the cruise ship I had a husband, son, and dog with me. The dog was like my dog in real life, but this dog was whole and healthy, unlike my dog that had been attacked by another dog and severely wounded. The cruise ship docked at a fancy resort area. My family was with the same group of people from the earlier excursion to the village. While we were shopping in the open market, one of the ladies from the ship was wading in the water along the beach. A large wave came ashore, engulfing her, and she was covered in brown, sticky seaweed.

Later that evening we were at a party at the resort and everyone was laughing and having a good time. The woman who had been covered in seaweed became suddenly ill and had red bumps all over her body. The ship's doctor took her away and put her in isolation until they could figure out what was making her sick. They finally determined she had some kind of fast-acting disease caused by bacteria from the seaweed. They sent all of the passengers back to the ship when other passengers started getting red bumps. Back on the ship, they took all of the sick people to an isolation area. They told the passengers that they could get a refund of their money for this trip or they could go on another trip for free. However, if they went on another trip they could not keep the items they bought while on this trip. The passengers had to decide between keeping the things they bought and getting a refund or get a future trip for free, but they could not have both. Most of the group were mad and said they certainly didn't ever want to go on another trip. I told them I had been on several cruises and I had never had any problems. This was just a rare occurrence.

My husband, son, dog, and I were all okay. However, I didn't sense it was really me, as if I was watching it all happen from outside. We headed back to our cabin. I was playing with the dog and feeling happy. Then I noticed a red spot under the dog's front leg. Soon my son and I also developed red spots.

Someone on the ship's crew told us they had information that my husband and I were not legally married because of some mix-up in the paperwork. My husband then became sick with red spots. We wanted to be officially married before we died, so we asked the captain of the ship to come and marry us in our cabin.

In real life my alarm went off, and I hit the snooze button and went back to sleep, falling back to the same place in the dream. When the last of our group on the ship died, it was like the movie Titanic. We were all together on the ship but not really alive. We could go anywhere we wanted and be dropped off to stay at any port. We went to a resort and the boys wanted to go to a gambling place. I said they didn't really need to go there, but they said it was what they wanted to do. I realized we would be split up and the idea made me uncomfortable, but I gave in and let them go. Then some girls from the ship went off to see some of the shops. My husband and I went for a walk along the beach.

Again, my alarm clock rang and I hit the snooze button and kept dreaming. My husband and I came back to the place where the boys were hanging out. They said they weren't happy there. The girls joined us and said they weren't happy either. We ended up going back to the ship with all the other people in the group who had died from the disease. No one had been happy in the places they chose to stay. We realized the place where everyone was happiest was with each other on the cruise ship.

The ship began to fill up with new people embarking on the next voyage. As I looked at the back of one of the new passengers, they turned around and, for an instant, their face changed to one of the people in our group. I realized our group would stay on the ship together forever.

## Interpretation

The first part of the dream at the school referred to various things going on in my life at that time. Not working on anything at the computer was a picture of how I felt unproductive at work.

I was also apprehensive about going back to school with younger students. So many things were changing with new technology. I felt as if I didn't belong at school, but stayed anyway. I was not engaging the change but hiding from it, not being confident in myself and my ability to learn new things. I was lost and uncertain about starting the veterinary assistant program.

The man who had lunch with me and helped me find my classes represented my therapist. He was helping me to get things straightened out in my mind and life and experience joy again.

The reference to not knowing how to swipe the card to pay for the food was about my feeling at odds with all the technological changes at work. There was training for a new software again, and I felt overwhelmed and incapable of learning it all.

The professor said that I had been missed in class. It felt wonderful to know that someone was expecting me and waiting for me. This was a picture of God waiting for me to come back to Him.

Having the wrong shoes for the hike symbolized being unprepared for the challenges ahead. It was a hard, unsure, uphill climb. I eventually got the right equipment (counseling) and at least began making steps to get out of depression, but it was slippery and easy to fall back. I had to tell myself it was okay to slide back down a little as long as I kept trying to go up the hill.

The cruise part of the dream was a symbol of the journey I was on. I was going with others, not alone. I had a sense of belonging to a group and the stability of a family.

The villagers using what they could find to make their products represented the ways I was making the money to pay for college for my husband and two daughters. I worked at my craft business on weekends and worked overtime at my job. I was the one working full-time and primarily providing for my family. I was isolated from the kind of life others had because it seemed like my whole life was spent working at my job and at home with no time left over for leisure activities.

The woman getting sick from the seaweed spoke to me that sometimes the waves of depression stir up the dirt at the bottom where I have stuffed it down. It can contaminate my relationships with others and keep me separated from other people.

The sick people were a picture of the unhealthy emotions I ignored through the busy life I lived. I did not want to face the truth that these emotions and the hectic pace of life were contributing to the sickness of depression. Losing those close to me represented the sense of loss and helplessness when I let go of the old habits and coping behavior that had been my crutch for so long.

The choice of a refund and keeping what you bought on the trip or a free trip in the future but giving up the things from the cruise meant I had to make a choice. I could go forward on another trip (keep seeking help for the depression) or keep the things accumulated on the trip (habits, processes, coping mechanisms, etc.) that I had carried with me all my life. I made a definite decision to go on another trip. I would not let one setback keep me from continuing on my journey.

All of the family being sick referred to all the emotions I was trying to sort out regarding my own family. I was dealing with the wounds of our dog from the attack, hurting for our children when life was hard for them, letting go of control in their lives, and not feeling close to Nick.

When I felt depressed, I pushed him away emotionally and physically. I looked whole and together in my outside appearance, but I was not on the inside. I struggled with my children going their own way and making their own choices. It hurt being apart from them. In the end, though, I let them be on their own.

However, Nick and I went forward together. The ship's captain coming to marry us was my affirmation deep inside that I was committed to do the hard work of regaining the closeness in our marriage.

The many interruptions from my alarm clock were bringing me closer to consciousness, but I felt a desperate need to finish the dream and have resolution to the things that were not making sense. The people were not happy with what they thought would make them happy. They were happiest when they were all together. It showed me that I needed to treasure and enjoy the times we are all together as a family instead of dwelling on missing them when we are apart. Family is what matters most.

## June 16, 2005—Wise Choices

I was going to a special concert with Nick and our daughter. They were late arriving at the theater, and I was very angry with both of them. I went ahead of them to find a seat near the front. Our daughter came up and sat beside me, but Nick went to sit up in the balcony. The concert began and the artist was James Taylor.

During intermission, we went outside and I told them I was sorry for being upset at them. We started back into the theater, when I noticed there was another show I had wanted to see playing at the theater across the street. I felt pulled between going back into the show with them or going across the street to the show I wanted to see. Nick said I needed to make my own decision. I chose James Taylor because the other show was going to be there for another month and I could see it later, but James Taylor was here only for one night.

## Interpretation

James Taylor is one of Nick's favorite singers. I wanted to see a different performance and Nick gave me a choice. Was I going to give in to what others wanted to do instead of standing up and saying what I wanted? Or was I going to be selfish and do what I wanted, no matter how it made them feel? Or was I going to show love by thinking of their desires, for a change, instead of everything being about me? Choosing to be with them and enjoying what they wanted to see was a sign of maturing and making progress in changing the self-centeredness caused by my depression and joining others enjoying special things.

## August 26, 2012—Acceptance of Job Changes

I was at my desk and working on some changes in a document when my boss came into the office. We joked around and talked about the events on the calendar for the day. He said there was a meeting with a very important client that morning and he wanted me to be with him in the meeting. I finished the changes to the document and pulled the file for the meeting from the file cabinet. After getting some coffee, I waited at the bank of six elevators to go up to the conference room. The buttons on the outside of the elevators were all mixed up, and I kept trying to catch an elevator that was going up, but they were all going down. I dashed from elevator to elevator, but the doors closed before I could get in them.

I finally got in an elevator that was going up, but when the doors opened, I was on the rooftop of the building. There were maintenance men working up there, and I asked them how to get back down to the offices. They showed me a different entrance to the elevator, and I got in and pushed the down button. However, it only went down a few floors and opened up in a different part of the building where there was a bakery selling cakes and cupcakes. I asked the sales clerk how to get back to the office building elevators, but she didn't know. I was beginning to panic because I was supposed to be in the meeting and it was almost time for it to begin. I walked around the corner and found another set of elevators. The door opened onto a ledge with a pole like a fire station. Two other people were in the elevator and they grabbed the pole and slid down. I couldn't see how far down the pole went, but there was no other way off the roof. I took hold of the pole and slid down in what felt like a free fall into nowhere. I eventually landed on the main floor, but the doorway next to the pole did not connect to the office building.

I went out into the street and walked around to the office part of the building, but the door was locked. I followed someone who had a key into the lobby. However, I did not have my ID badge with me and the security guards would not let me into the elevator area. I thought of calling someone I knew to have them come down and get me, but I couldn't think of anyone to call. I was finally able to sneak into the elevator area in the middle of a group of people. When I got in the elevator, the button for my floor was missing. I pushed the button for the floor below mine, thinking I would take the internal stairs up one flight.

When I finally arrived on my floor, I walked around the halls, but I couldn't find my desk. All the desks were gone and there were box-shaped machines sitting everywhere. One of the security guards asked me what I was doing there and I told him I was looking for my desk. In the hallway there were two other women, and one of them said the company was getting rid of everyone. I went looking for my boss, but I couldn't find his office either. I asked the guard where my boss was and he said my boss no longer worked at the company. He then took the three of us women to a room that had an opening like a laundry chute and pushed each one of us into the chute. We were being discarded like the trash, with no value.

## Interpretation

The initial confusion with the elevators demonstrates the confusion I felt about my new career as a veterinary assistant and trying to find my way after twenty-five years as a secretary and paralegal in a law office. It also was part of the grieving process of leaving a job and bosses that I liked and entering something unknown. Being up on the rooftop was a picture of how vulnerable I felt. I knew very little about my new job and had to learn different skills as I went.

Coming out onto a ledge was representative of losing my new job after only seven months because I broke my foot. I felt stranded again, with only one way out, but it was like free-falling into uncertainty. I did not know what kind of job I could find now or how we would manage financially if I didn't find work soon.

Not being able to get back into the building and no longer having my job was a picture of coming to grips with the reality that I could not work as a veterinary assistant any longer because my foot could not take the stress of standing for ten hours a day. It was about accepting the fact that the door to what I thought was a new career was closed and I had no place there anymore.

The laundry chute illustrated my feelings of being dumped with no dignity or value because I was broken. I could not do this job anymore and I did not want to go back to the stress of a law office. I felt useless and incapable of handling any kind of job. My self-confidence was almost nonexistent, and I was afraid I had been out of an office environment for so long that I would not be current enough on technology to be hired by anyone.

## May 9, 2011—Admitting Feelings about the Past

I was in a foreign country that was very tropical and staying with a family who were missionaries. They had several children and a dog that looked like my dog in real life. Sometimes you could hear animals such as gorillas, elephants, and tigers fighting in the jungle, which was not too far from their house. One side of their house didn't seem to have a wall; it just opened to the jungle.

There were also pythons and small poisonous snakes. Once a python had their little boy, and I ran and poked the snake with a stick until it let go of the boy. Another time a different snake came near their house and bit the little dog on his back and then slithered away. The boy and I raced to pick up the dog. He was already stiff and paralyzed from the venom. I held the dog, cradled like a baby, and told it I was sorry we didn't get there in time. The little boy hugged his dog and said he loved it and then it died.

Shortly thereafter, the little boy said he didn't want to live here anymore; he wanted to go home. His parents said they couldn't leave right then. The little boy ran away and everyone was looking all over the village for him. I found him in the upstairs of a grist mill on the outskirts of town. He asked me not to tell anyone where he was hiding. I didn't tell anyone, but I brought him food and water. One day his father was out searching for him and saw the boy outside the mill. He ran to the boy and hugged him, tears running down his face. He told his son that he was sorry for not realizing how upset he was about losing his dog, and they went home together.

Later that week I was visiting neighbors down the road from the little boy. They had a cocker spaniel and it had just given birth to seven puppies. I went over to see the puppies, and I saw a big black dog running toward me, bearing its teeth and growling. Since there were several black puppies in the litter, I realized he must be the father. When he was about five feet from me, I held up my hand and told him to sit, looking him straight in the eye. He stopped and sat down. I continued talking to him in a slow, calming voice and told him I was not going to hurt his puppies. I started to approach him slowly with my hand extended as I talked. As I got up next to him, I let him sniff my hand and asked him if he wanted to see his puppies. I asked one of the neighbors to pick up one of the black puppies slowly and hand it to me behind my back. As I continued to talk to the black dog, I brought the puppy around front and said, "Here is one of your little ones." He sniffed it in my hand and then licked the puppy. I put the puppy on the ground and it scampered off to its mom and snuggled up next to her to nurse with the other puppies. The big dog looked at me and I told him it was okay and that he could go to them. He looked from me to them and back to me and then trotted over to the mom and puppies.

I went into the house with the owners and in the corner of the kitchen was a dog that was the same breed as the one the little boy lost. I asked the people if I could give that dog to the little boy, and they said they would love for him to have the dog. I went back to the missionaries' house and told the little boy I had a surprise for him. He was overjoyed with his new dog.

The parents told me they were returning home because they realized they needed to spend more time focusing on the needs of their children. They were all packed up and had everything loaded on the boat. Everyone in the village went to the dock to see them off. Two of their children were not on the boat and I went to look for them. I found them looking at toys in one of the market stalls. I grabbed them up and ran to the water, but the boat had already pulled away from the dock and was quite a distance from shore. The parents shouted that the boat could not return to the dock. They asked me to bring the two children to them on the next boat that left in three weeks. I promised I would bring them home.

Suddenly, a man from the village came running up to the dock and said several men had been up in the hills hunting and they saw the lions congregated together on a hill on one side of the valley and they were acting very aggressive. On the other side of the valley, they saw a herd of wildebeest all stirred up because of the lions and they were ready to stampede. He said both the wildebeest and the lions would reach the village by the next morning and everyone needed to make preparations to keep safe.

## Interpretation

The little boy running away and "wanting to go home" was like a subconscious desire to escape my life with my dad, even though at that young age I didn't know what it was really like there. I did leave and go back to live with my mom, but the hurt from being separated from my dad went with me.

The part about the big dog and the puppies showed how I felt around animals. I had a way of being with them and working to help them not be afraid. I think it also portrays my desire to make things right in reuniting the family, the way I wanted to reunite mine. The two children left behind symbolized my dad being left behind when I went back to my mom, only he never came back to us. Bringing joy to the boy with the new dog was about being able to find joy in giving to others again. I felt like I finally had something of value to offer to others.

The parents returning to spend time with their children represented when my mom and I moved from the city out to the suburbs. It was supposed to be different and better for me and in most ways it was. I had friends to play with in our neighborhood and attended a good school. But that was also the place where the incidents with Mom and Ben occurred and I received the message that I didn't really belong. I sensed I had been emotionally left behind by Mom, like the parents left their children behind. I was on my own and had to take care of myself. However, as I promised the parents in the dream that I would bring the children back to them, I eventually learned from the Bible and other Christians who took me under their wing that God promised He would be with me and take care of me. One day He will bring me home to Himself in Heaven forever.

The reference to the lions and wildebeest on either side of the valley ready to come into the village represented the war going on inside of me. I knew what the Bible said about immorality was right, but I struggled with the fact that what Mom was doing was wrong. I felt angry with her for doing something that was against what God said, and yet she was my mom and I loved her. I didn't know how to reconcile the two opposing truths. Ultimately, I accepted the reality that I had no control over her choices, even though they affected my life. She had to answer to God for her lifestyle and she endured some hurtful consequences. Eventually, she sought and received God's forgiveness.

I was still responsible for honoring my mom as Scripture commanded and complying with her wishes while I was under her roof. But I also was seeking to follow God's plan for my life and be obedient to what His Word said about how to live my life, including forgiving my mom.

# 10

# Freedom in Christ

One night a few years ago, God woke me up and began speaking to me, telling me to write down what He was saying. I got up and got some paper and a pen and started writing down all the things that were running through my head. God said I was to share what He had given me before the congregation at my church. It had been quite a long time since I had sensed God speaking to me as clearly as He did that night. I'd like to share the main part of what I said at church about freedom in Christ and demonstrate how God used the lyrics of a song to help me see that my Heavenly Father is not the same as my earthly father and that I needed to forgive my dad. Although I was nervous about sharing and being so vulnerable in front of so many people, I did it out of obedience, believing God had someone there who needed to hear this message.

Several years ago I was at a concert and heard a song that God used as a turning point in my life. The song is by Mark Schulz and is titled, "You Are a Child of Mine." Let me share a little of why this song had such an impact on me and how some of the lyrics express the same truths I discovered in the Bible. All of my life I have struggled with the concept of God as my Heavenly Father. I imagined God was like my earthly father. I became a Christian when I was seventeen, but all my life I compartmentalized God into the roles of Jesus as Savior, the Holy Spirit living inside me, and God as Creator but never as Father. I thought God, like my earthly father, could not be trusted to protect me, provide for me, or care what happens to me. If He did, how could He have let things happen to a defenseless child like me?

The main message of Mark Schulz's song is about our being God's child and the freedom we have in Christ through that relationship. God helped me to understand that He is perfect love and He created me in His image.

"Freedom in Christ"—what does that mean? I want to look at two aspects of the freedom we have been given through Christ's death and His payment for our sins.[2] The first aspect is that we have obtained freedom **from** certain things.

## Freedom from Sin and the Law

One of the most obvious freedoms is the freedom from sin and the law. In Romans 6:18 we read, "You have been

---

[2]    For a complete list of Scripture, see the index at the end of this book.

set free from sin and have become slaves of righteousness."[3] Also in the New Testament we read that Jesus sets us free from the law of sin and death. Colossians states, "For he has rescued us from the dominion of darkness and brought us into the kingdom of the Son he loves, in whom we have redemption, the forgiveness of sins."

## Freedom from Lies

Sometimes we overlook other things from which we have been given freedom. One is freedom from the lies of Satan and others that pervert our perception of who we are in Christ. In 1 Peter 5:8 we are told, "Your enemy the devil prowls around like a roaring lion looking for someone to devour," and in Job we see how Satan attacks and accuses us when Satan asks God, "Does Job fear God for nothing? You have put a hedge around him and everything he has. But stretch out your hand and strike everything he has and he will curse you to your face."

Satan was at work in the beginning at the garden, putting doubt in Eve's mind that "surely you will not die." In Matthew 4 we read of Satan's temptation of Jesus. Satan tried to trap Jesus with fleshly appetites (food—turn the stone into bread), power (quoting Scripture to tempt Jesus—jump from the mountain, the angels will come and bear you up), and idolatry and false worship (giving Jesus everything in the world in exchange for denying God).

---

[3]    All Scripture is taken from The Holy Bible, New International Version, (New York: New York International Bible Society, 1978).

Colossians says, "Once you were alienated from God and were enemies in your minds because of your evil behavior. But now he has reconciled you by Christ's physical body through death to present you holy in his sight, without blemish and free from accusation." We no longer stand as those who are condemned by our sins, but forgiven by the blood of Christ.

## Freedom from the World's Mind-set

We get caught up in thinking like the world thinks. We forget this world is not our home. In 1 Peter 2:9 we read, "But you are a chosen people, a royal priesthood, a holy nation, a people belonging to God that you may declare the praises of him who called you out of darkness and into his wonderful light. Once you were not a people, but now you are a people." Ephesians tells us we are fellow citizens of God's people and members of God's household. Elsewhere in the New Testament God tells us how we can have freedom in our minds and thoughts by not conforming to the ways of this world, but being changed by the renewing of our minds.

## Freedom from Fear

Through our freedom in Christ, we are also free from fear. In Matthew 6:25-34 Jesus tells the people, "Don't worry about the material things of this world. Your Father in Heaven knows you need them. Seek first His kingdom and He will provide them." Paul reminds us that God shall supply all your needs through His riches in Christ Jesus. John says perfect love casts out fear. Finally, we read in 2 Timothy 1:7, "God did not give us a spirit of fear, but a spirit of power, of love and of self-discipline." God wants us to be free from fear and live in the hope that our life in Christ gives us. To live free from fear is a choice we must make every day.

## Freedom from Our Past

One of the most important freedoms we have gained in our relationship with God is freedom from our past. When we become Christians, God makes us new and works to conform us to the image of Christ. Second Corinthians 5:17 says, "Therefore, if anyone is in Christ, he is a new creation; the old has gone and the new has come." The New Testament also lets us know that God made you alive in Christ.

This freedom does not mean that we will not suffer consequences for choices we made in our past. But through this new life in Christ, we have freedom from our past shaping, dictating, and controlling the way we think, speak, and act. We no longer have to live according to the old messages and lies we have heard.

## Freedom from Guilt and Shame

We are free from the guilt and shame of things we have done that have been forgiven by the blood of Christ! First John 1:9 tells us, "If we confess our sins, he is faithful and just and will forgive us our sins and purify us from all unrighteousness." David says in the Psalms that God has removed our sins from us as far as the east is from the west. Once those sins are confessed and forgiven by God, there is no need for us to feel shame or guilt about them. They are covered by Christ's blood and God sees us as spotless and pure! Satan is the one who brings those things to our mind to make us feel guilty or ashamed so that we stay shackled in bondage to those things to make us ineffective in our Christian walk. We need to see ourselves as God sees us and forgive ourselves as God has forgiven us.

The lyrics of Mark Schulz's song say,[4] "I've been hearing voices telling me that I can never be what I want to be. Haunting me at night and saying there is nothing to believe. When I am alone at night, that is when I hear the lie, you'll never be enough." We cannot deal with guilt and shame by ourselves and in our own strength. That is why we need to be part of the local Body of Christ, the church, so we have others to walk alongside us through difficult times. God certainly can help us, but sometimes He works through other people to be instruments of His healing and peace.

We so often get those tapes stuck in our head: You can't serve God or do anything for God because you used to do or be _____ (fill in the blank); you will never be good enough; God couldn't love YOU after what you have done. These are all lies from the pit of hell. God can change us so we do not operate out of our past. He is molding us and making us into the image of Christ, through whom we can

---

4    © 2003 Crazy Romaine Music (ASCAP) (Administered by Music Services) / Here's To Jo Music (BMI) All Rights Reserved. Used by permission.

do and be anything. God wants to erase those tapes and put in our minds His truth about who we are—we are free in Christ, joint heirs with Jesus, children of God!

Romans 8:15-17 says, "The Spirit himself testifies with our spirit that we are God's children. If we are children, then we are heirs, heirs of God and co-heirs with Christ." Galatians reminds us that we are all sons of God through faith in Christ Jesus, and since you are a son, God has made you also an heir. Ephesians and 1 John say the Gentiles are heirs together with Israel, members of one body, and sharers in the promise in Christ and God showed His love by calling us the children of God.

Living in freedom from our past is a choice we must make every day. The lyrics say,[5] "So I listen as you tell me who I am and who it is that I'm gonna be, and I hang on every word, knowing I have heard I am yours and I am free. Though I'm giving into fear, *if I listen* I can hear you say" the truth of who I am. I am a child of God (emphasis mine)!

With this freedom, God has a plan for our lives. In the Psalms David says that God will fulfill his purposes for me and I was made in the secret place. All the days ordained for me were written in your book before one of them came to be. In the New Testament Paul says God, who began a good work in you, will carry it on to completion until the day of Christ Jesus. A verse that has meant a lot to Nick and me as a promise from God is Jeremiah 29:11: "For I know the plans I have for you, declares the Lord, plans to prosper you and not to harm you, plans to give you hope

---

[5] © 2003 Crazy Romaine Music (ASCAP) (Administered by Music Services) / Here's To Jo Music (BMI) All Rights Reserved. Used by permission.

and a future." This has been a guiding verse as we have faced tough decisions in our life together.

Now I'd like to talk about the second aspect of our freedom in Christ. It not only frees us from things; it frees us **to** things.

## Freedom to Be Loved by God

One of these is the freedom to be loved by God. I struggle to wrap my emotions around this concept. I know in my head and my heart that God loves me, but I find it hard to feel God's love sometimes.

In Jeremiah 31:3 God says, "I have loved you with an everlasting love; I have drawn you with lovingkindness." In the New Testament Jesus tells us that He loves us the same way the Father loves Him. Romans gives us a beautiful picture of God's love for us because Christ died for us while we were still sinners. We didn't have to clean ourselves up or get our act together before God would love us. Later in Romans, Paul talks about all the things that cannot separate us from the love of God, and in John 3:16 and 1 John 3:16, respectively, we read about God's love for us: "For God so loved the world [and us individually] that he gave his only son, that whoever believes on him should not perish but have eternal life (emphasis mine)," and, "This is how we know what love is: Jesus Christ laid down his life for us."

When we let our lives be controlled by guilt and shame, we believe that others could not possibly love us. We hold them at arm's length and don't let them get too close. If they see the real me, they couldn't love me. But God says He loves us just as we are right now, even if we are far away from Him.

## Freedom to Be Loved by Others

The second thing we have freedom to do is to be loved by others. I learned what love is from Nick. He knew my background of abuse, neglect, and abandonment and he still loved me. Because of my experiences, my concept of marital relations was as an unpleasant duty to be endured by a wife. Nick was so patient and loving, being content with whatever I was able to give and not demanding more. When God freed me of my misconceptions about intimacy in marriage, I could truly see the love and sacrifice Nick had made for me.

## Freedom to Love Others

When we embrace being loved by God and others, we are also free to love others as God loves us. In Matthew 22:37-39 we read, "No greater love has a man than this, that he would lay down his life for another." When we feel secure in God's love and our true position as His child, we can express His love to the unlovely, broken, and wounded around us. Jesus told the crowd in Matthew 26:35-40, "When I was naked you clothed me, when I was hungry you fed me, when I was in prison you visited me." We are free to love those around us who are sometimes the outcast and shunned in society with God's love and compassion.

## Freedom to Give

The freedom to love others also connects us to another freedom—we are free to give. We can give of our time, our money, our resources, and ourselves to bring the Gospel and the Kingdom of Heaven to lost souls here on earth. Giving can come in many forms—delivering meals on wheels, writing a note of encouragement to someone going through a tough time, making dinner for someone who is sick, giving above your tithe to a ministry that is helping people in other parts of the world, sharing your story with someone or going on a mission trip.

## Freedom to Be Healed

Another freedom we have is the freedom to be healed. When we were lost sinners, sin could not heal us from the separation with God. In Genesis 2 and 3, we see that spiritual death was the result of Adam and Eve's sin in the garden. But in 1 Corinthians 15:21 we see that "as in Adam all die, through Christ all shall be made alive." Only through our belief and acceptance of the work of Jesus shedding His blood on the cross as payment for our sin can we be healed from the hurts and scars of sin. David says in the Psalms that I will be whiter than snow if I let God wash away the stain of sin. He cries out to God to "have mercy on me and heal me, for I have sinned against you." Isaiah 53:5 speaks of the coming Messiah and says, "But he was pierced for our transgressions, he was crushed for our iniquities; the punishment that brought us peace was upon him, and by his wounds we are healed."

When we become children of God, we can allow God into the dark corners of our lives where we hide the hurts, disappointments, fears, misery, hatred, etc., and let Him begin the healing process of banishing those areas from our life, if we choose to let Him. The process can be long and painful, but God does not abandon us. He is with us in each step of the process. My favorite passage is Isaiah 43:1-3, which says, "This is what the Lord says—he who created you O Jacob, who formed you O Israel, fear not, for I have redeemed you; I have summoned you by name, you are mine. When you pass *through* the waters, I will be with you; when you pass *through* the rivers, they will not sweep over you. When you walk *through* the fire, you will not be burned; the flames will not harm you. For I am the Lord your God, the Holy One of Israel, your Savior (emphasis mine)." God does not always save us from trials and troubles in our lives, but He always walks through them with us and we will come out on the other side. God wants to heal us from physical, emotional, and spiritual wounds and scars. It is up to us to allow Him into those sensitive and painful areas of our lives.

## Freedom to Forgive

A very important thing we are given freedom to do is forgive. But we must remember that the standard of forgiveness is as God has forgiven you, so you should forgive others. One of the things that I have found important in my journey with God is that not only must we forgive others but we must forgive ourselves, as I talked about earlier, in order to be free from guilt and shame.

# 11

# Forgiveness and Healing

## Forgiving My Father

Through time in prayer and studying the Bible, I realized that I had to forgive my father to be in right relationship with God. I could not be close to God while harboring anger in my heart against my father. One of the tools I used to help me forgive my dad was writing a letter to him to say the things I never got a chance to say face-to-face. I closed that letter with the following:

> I want you to know I am letting go of the anger, hate and sadness I have always felt towards you. I have come to a place where I can understand some of your reasons for the choices you made and I forgive you for the things that happened when I was little. But

most of all, I am really sad that you missed so much of my life, my wonderful husband, your grandchildren, and that you never knew what kind of person God helped me to become.

## Forgiving God

I know this will sound strange, but sometimes it is even necessary for us to forgive God because we hold grudges, anger, or resentment towards Him. As I said earlier, I was angry with God for what I perceived as Him not being there for me, not protecting me, etc. I could not trust Him to guide my life. God doesn't need to be forgiven by us, but we need to forgive Him for our own sake to clear away any walls we have built up between God and ourselves. I do not think it is wrong to argue with God or be angry with Him about a situation. He is big enough to take anything we can say to Him. He would rather we be honest with Him than stuff those feelings inside and let them fester into bitterness. He knows them anyway. But our expression of them out loud to Him helps us heal.

I now know that God was there with me as a child and He did protect me. It could have been so much worse. Abused children usually take one of three paths: They go into prostitution, they become abusers themselves, or they seek therapy and healing for the trauma. God, in His love and mercy, spared me from further harm and brought me on a journey to healing.

As I struggled through this process of my perception of God and the truth of who He really is, I told Him in a journal entry that I was tired of "playing church," going through the motions, saying all the right words so everyone would think I was spiritual, when inside I was as dry as dust. I told Him if He didn't show up and be real in my life, I was done. I was walking away from church and having nothing else to do with Him.

God did show up! He is ALWAYS faithful to meet us when we sincerely cry out to Him. That next week I went to the Mark Schulz concert and heard the song. I bought the CD and played it over and over and over again, hearing the truth of what it meant for God to be my Father and for me to be His child. I heard Him tell me that He designed me uniquely and that He has made me free in Christ to be a child of His. That night God put me on a path to bring healing in my life, freeing me from fears of abandonment and provision, and along the way I learned to trust Him for everything in my life. When I was able to see the truth of who God really was and that I am His child and a joint heir with Christ, I learned that I can appropriate all that is God's through His Spirit living in me. Through this proper relationship as His child, I have access to all the resources I need to live in the freedom Christ purchased on the cross. I know God can heal each of you from whatever you are struggling with, if you will allow Him to do it in His way and time. He loves you more than you can ever imagine and truly wants what is best for you. I offer this prayer for you and hope you will listen to God speak His truth to your heart.

Abba Father, thank you for showing me Your unconditional love that is not based on my performance or how good I am but because You created me uniquely for a love relationship with You. Thank You that You have given me the freedom and grace to forgive my father, myself, and You and that You have brought healing to my wounded heart. May Your Spirit speak Your truth to those who read this, the truth of who You created them to be and help them to live in the freedom You gave us through Christ's death, which was Your ultimate expression of love. Amen.

# Epilogue

One night about eleven years after I began seeing my therapist, I had a wonderful dream. I was attending a high school reunion and Scott was there. We talked about our families and what was going on in our lives. Then he said he had to go. I told him I understood, that it was time for him to leave. He said he would always be close by if I needed him. I gave him a hug goodbye and then realized the little girl was standing by my side. She looked up at me with questioning eyes. I knelt down, scooped her into my arms, and hugged her tightly. As I stood up, I told her it was okay for her to go with Scott because he would keep her safe. She smiled, took his hand, and they walked out of the building.

I have never had another of what I call my "therapy dreams" since that last dream. It was as if God were saying the hardest part was over and I could now move forward with the mature and healthy emotions of an adult. There would still be attitudes and memories I would need to confront to maintain my emotional well-being but not to the same depth of revelation and pain that I had come through.

Although this journey of depression was very difficult and, at times, I wanted to give up, I am so very grateful that God cared about me and He loved me enough to take me through this process of redemption, relieving the depth of my depression. He showed me how to let go of the anger and hurt that had bound and strangled me for so long and how to forgive others and myself. May He do the same for you!

# Scripture Index

Romans 6:18—You have been set free from sin and have become slaves of righteousness.

Romans 8:2—Through Christ Jesus the law of the Spirit of life set me free from the law of sin and death.

Galatians 5:1—It is for freedom that Christ has set us free.

Colossians 1:13—For he has rescued us from the dominion of darkness and brought us into the kingdom of the Son he loves, in whom we have redemption, the forgiveness of sins.

1 Peter 5:8—Your enemy the devil prowls around like a roaring lion looking for someone to devour.

Job 1:9-11—Does Job fear God for nothing? … Have you not put a hedge around him and his household and everything he has? … But stretch out your hand and strike everything he has and he will curse you to your face.

Genesis 3:4—Satan at work in the garden putting doubt in Eve's mind that "you will not surely die."

Colossians 1:21-22—Once you were alienated from God and were enemies in your minds because of your evil behavior. But now he has reconciled you by Christ's physical body through death to present you holy in his sight, without blemish and free from accusation.

1 Peter 2:9—But you are a chosen people, a royal priesthood, a holy nation, a people belonging to God, that you may declare the praises of him who called you out of darkness into his wonderful light. Once you were not a people, but now you are the people of God.

Ephesians 2:19—You are no longer foreigners and aliens, but fellow citizens with God's people and members of God's household.

Romans 12:2—Do not conform any longer to the pattern of this world, but be transformed by the renewing of your mind.

Matthew 6:31-34—So don't worry, saying, "What shall we eat?" or "What shall we drink?" or "What shall we wear?" … Your heavenly Father knows you need them. But seek first his kingdom and his righteousness and all these things will be given to you as well.

Philippians 4:19—My God will meet all your needs according to his glorious riches in Christ Jesus.

1 John 4:18—There is no fear in love. But perfect love drives out fear.

2 Timothy 1:7—For God did not give us a spirit of fear, but a spirit of power, of love and of self-discipline.

2 Corinthians 5:17—Therefore, if anyone is in Christ, he is a new creation; the old has gone, the new has come!

Colossians 2:13—When you were dead in your sins and in the uncircumcision of your sinful nature, God made you alive in Christ.

1 John 1:9—If we confess our sins, he is faithful and just and will forgive us our sins and purify us from all unrighteousness.

Psalm 103:12—As far as the east is from the west, so far has he removed our transgressions from us.

Philippians 4:13—I can do everything through Christ who gives me strength.

Romans 8:16-17—The Spirit himself testifies with our spirit that we are God's children. Now if we are children, then we are heirs, heirs of God and co-heirs with Christ.

Galatians 3:26—You are all sons of God through faith in Christ Jesus.

Galatians 4:7—So you are no longer a slave but a son; and since you are a son, God has made you also an heir.

Ephesians 3:6—Through the Gospel the Gentiles are heirs together with Israel, members of one body, and sharers together in the promise in Christ Jesus.

1 John 3:1—How great is the love the Father has lavished on us, that we should be called children of God.

Psalm 138:8—The Lord will fulfill his purpose for me; your love, O Lord, endures forever.

Psalm 139:15-16My frame was not hidden from you when I was made in the secret place…. All the days ordained for me were written in your book before one of them came to be.

Philippians 1:6—Being confident of this, that he who began a good work in you will carry it on to completion until the day of Christ Jesus.

Jeremiah 29:11—For I know the plans I have for you, declares the Lord, plans to prosper you and not to harm you, plans to give you hope and a future.

Jeremiah 31:3—I have loved you with an everlasting love; I have drawn you with lovingkindness.

John 15:9—As the Father has loved me, so have I loved you. Now remain in my love.

Romans 5:8—But God demonstrates his own love for us in this: While we were yet sinners, Christ died for us.

Romans 8:38-39—For I am convinced that neither death nor life, neither angels nor demons, neither the present nor the future, nor any powers, neither height nor depth, nor anything else in all creation, will be able to separate us from the love of God that is in Christ Jesus our Lord.

Ephesians 2:4-5—But because of his great love for us, God, who is rich in mercy, made us alive with Christ even when we were dead in sin, it is by grace you have been saved.

John 3:16—For God so loved the world that he gave his one and only son, that whoever believes in him shall not perish but have eternal life.

1 John 3:16—This is how we know what love is: Jesus Christ laid down his life for us.

John 15:13—Greater love has no man than this, that he lay down his life for his friends.

Matthew 25:35-36—For I was hungry and you gave me something to eat, I was thirsty and you gave me something to drink, I was a stranger and you invited me in, I needed clothes and you clothed me, I was sick and you looked after me, I was in prison and you cane to visit me.

1 Corinthians 15:22—For as in Adam all die, so in Christ all will be made alive.

Psalm 51:7—Wash me, and I will be whiter than snow.

Psalm 41:4—I said, O Lord, have mercy on me; heal me, for I have sinned against you.

Isaiah 1:18—Though your sins are like scarlet, they shall be as white as snow, though they are red as crimson, they shall be like wool.

Isaiah 53:5—But he was pierced for our transgressions, he was crushed for our iniquities; the punishment that brought us peace was upon him, and by his wounds we are healed.

Isaiah 43:1-3—But now, this is what the Lord says—he who created you, O Jacob, who formed you, O Israel: Fear not, for I have redeemed you; I have summoned you by name; you are mine. When you pass *through* the waters, I will be with you; when you pass *through* the rivers, they will not sweep over you. When you walk *through* the fire, you will not be burned; the flames will not set you ablaze. For I am the Lord, your God, the Holy One of Israel, your Savior (emphasis mine).

# About the Author

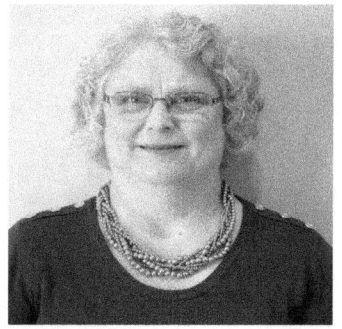

A nita Placido works as a bank teller in Wilmore, Kentucky. She lives with her husband, Nick and their black lab, Lacy. She has two daughters, Sarah and Miriam, and two son-in-laws, Jack and José, plus three grandchildren, Katharine, Rachel and Samuel. She loves to crochet, cook and read mystery novels in her spare time.

www.ingramcontent.com/pod-product-compliance
Lightning Source LLC
Chambersburg PA
CBHW060522130626
46553CB00002B/610